Advance Praise for *Riptide*

"I defy any therapist to read Barbara Hale-Seubert's book and remain emotionally aloof. While written as a personal story, *Riptide* will benefit anyone who is dealing with a mentally ill or addicted family member. It serves as a model for how to go through such an experience with honesty and presence, while showing others how to care for oneself throughout the process. In writing about such a loss, Barbara beautifully details the pains, frustrations, guilt, anger, and even joys of her journey. She writes with genuine authenticity, warmth, compassion, and forgiveness — certainly for her daughter, and finally, for herself."

—David Mandelbaum, Ph.D., family therapist

"Barbara Hale-Seubert has captured something I've never seen someone do in writing: the rawness and genuine authenticity of a mother's pain. In the course of her book, she unlocked that pain and gave mothers permission to acknowledge their own needs and reactions."

—Carolyn Hodges, CEO of the Nutrition Clinic
and Sol Stone Center for Eating Disorders

"Barbara Hale-Seubert takes us on a compelling, heart-wrenching journey into her family's fatal ten-year odyssey. Miraculously, Barbara is able to tell her devastating story in a way that provides hope and guidance to others. There are many families out there who need the direction and reassurance that *Riptide* provides: they are not alone in their struggles and they should not be blamed."

—Doris Smeltzer, author of *Andrea's Voice: Silenced by Bulimia*

"Barbara Hale-Seubert's raw honesty opens the door for others to walk through. She gives us a space to feel — free of judgment — and a place to honor our pain. In doing so she gives us hope. By sharing her and Erin's journey, she joins us in ours."

—Mary Ellen Clausen, executive director of Ophelia's Place

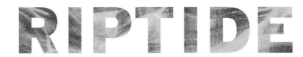

RIPTIDE

RIPTIDE

STRUGGLING WITH AND RESURFACING
FROM A DAUGHTER'S EATING DISORDER

Barbara Hale-Seubert

ECW Press

Published by ECW Press
2120 Queen Street East, Suite 200, Toronto, Ontario, Canada M4E 1E2
416.694.3348 / info@ecwpress.com

LIBRARY AND ARCHIVES CANADA CATALOGUING IN PUBLICATION

Hale-Seubert, Barbara
Riptide : struggling with and resurfacing from a daughter's eating disorder / Barbara Hale-Seubert.

ISBN 978-1-55022-995-0
ALSO ISSUED AS:
978-1-55490-906-3 (PDF); 978-1-55490-969-8 (EPUB)

1. Hale-Seubert, Barbara. 2. Erin Leah, 1976–2000. 3. Eating disorders in adolescence—Patients—Family relationships —United States. 4. Eating disorders in adolescence—Patients— United States—Biography. 5. Anorexia nervosa—Patients—United States—Biography. 6. Bulimia—Patients—United States—Biography. 7. Psychotherapists—United States—Biography. 1. Title.

RJ506.E18H34 2011   618.92'85260092   C2010-906829-7

Developing editor: Jen Hale
Cover and Text Design: Tania Craan
Typesetting: Mary Bowness
Printing: Friesens   1   2   3   4   5

To the best of her ability, the author has recreated experiences, places, people, and organizations from her memories of them. In order to protect the privacy of others she has, in some instances, changed the names of certain people and details of events and places.

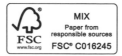

MIX
Paper from
responsible sources
FSC® C016245

PRINTED AND BOUND IN CANADA

ECW PRESS
ecwpress.com

To Erin Leah

My first true love

CONTENTS

FOREWORD

MARGO MAINE, Ph.D, FAED

Statistics are people with the tears wiped away.

Countless journal articles and books are devoted to the heartbreaking statistics ushered into people's lives by devastating eating disorders. An Amazon search reveals nearly 30,000 books available through its website alone. This growing literature is full of faceless statistics warning us that eating disorders are affecting more and more people of all ages, from young children to senior citizens, of every race, socio-economic status, ethnicity, and gender, and in more than 40 countries worldwide. It describes the challenges of treatment and the unanswered research questions about its effectiveness. *Riptide: Struggling with and Resurfacing from a Daughter's Eating Disorder* gets away from the numbers and puts a face on the problem — a face weeping with heartbreak.

Nothing is worse than the gut-wrenching pain parents experience when watching their child suffer. This pain is magnified exponentially when "the child" is no longer a child and the problem is psychiatric, as the answers of diagnosis, treatment, and a path to recovery are all so elusive. There is no lullaby nor Band-Aid, no quick fix nor clarity about how to help in these situations. Although physical illness is itself a challenge to the sufferer and family, usually the treatment options and resources are mapped out and people are able to talk about the problem and receive support. Not so when the diagnosis is psychiatric, or even more complicated, as eating disorders are, spanning both the psychiatric and physical worlds.

Eating disorders are what we call biopsychosocial problems, as they have roots in each area and manifest themselves in each realm: the biological, the psychological, and the social. They have the highest morbidity and mortality rate of all psychiatric illnesses. Even the afflicted who receive good treatment and have family support along the way may end up succumbing to the ravages of these disorders. When families first encounter the diagnosis, many feel instantly overwhelmed and defeated, while others work hard to remain optimistic that their child will beat the odds. In every case, the suffering is immense, and, all too often, it's compounded by a lack of understanding and compassion, in both professional and personal relationships. It can be overwhelming.

Eating disorders, at least temporarily, create a cloud or a fog around the sufferer. Once it begins, the disorder seems to have a life of its own, as starvation creates an obsession with food, emotions are translated into the language of fat, self-esteem and self-image are destroyed, and personal identity becomes wrapped around the illusion of control found in eating-disordered behaviors. I have come to see the eating disorder as a life preserver — one that my patients truly feel they will drown without. The goal of treatment and the key to survival is to develop other resources to avoid that powerful feeling of terror patients experience when they believe others are trying to take their life preserver away.

For loved ones, especially parents, one of the greatest challenges brought on by eating disorders is to stay connected with this person (usually female), who now is only a shadow of her self and who rails against any efforts to break down the barrier of the eating disorder, just as anyone thrashes to hold onto a life preserver when she fears drowning. As a clinician who has specialized in treating eating disorders for the past three decades, I, too, struggle at times to stay connected, to manage my anxiety about their condition and about the likelihood I will penetrate the fog before it totally destroys her and she loses her life. I can only imagine what parents feel, as I see the pain, the confusion, the disillusionment, the guilt, and the self-doubt in my office each day.

In *Riptide: Struggling with and Resurfacing from a Daughter's Eating Disorder*, Barabara Hale-Seubert discloses the painful struggle she experienced as the mother of a young woman who suffered and succumbed to an eating disorder. She offers no easy answers, but uses her own experience to help other families to cope with the emotional riptides and consequences of this illness. Her path was complicated by her professional role as a therapist, who was capable of helping so many people overcome the issues that brought them to her door, but often felt inept with her own daughter. Her strength, courage, and soul-baring honesty are amazing, as is her hope to enable other parents to survive the riptide and avoid drowning themselves. It is this kind of self-examination and brutal honesty that will get eating disorders out of the closets of shame and embarrassment and into the light of hope, understanding, and healing.

Despite the tragic loss of her daughter Erin, Barbara Hale-Seubert has found a way past her tears and heartbreak to find meaning, connection, and renewal. She shows us that facing pain is the only way through it, and that time helps to heal the weary souls of parents who have experienced a child's life-threatening illness. Although prompted to write because of Erin's death, Barbara is truly writing about life, embracing both her daughter's and her own, in all their complexity. If a story can be profoundly sad, but inspirational at the same time, *Riptide: Struggling with and Resurfacing from a Daughter's Eating Disorder* is that story.

An expert in the treatment of eating disorders for nearly three decades, Dr. Margo Maine is the editor of *Effective Clinical Practice in the Treatment of Eating Disorders: The Heart of the Matter* (with Davis and Shure), and the author of *The Body Myth: Adult Women and the Pressure to Be Perfect* (with Joe Kelly), *Father Hunger: Fathers, Daughters and the Pursuit of Thinness*; and *Body Wars: Making Peace with Women's Bodies*. She is a senior editor of *Eating Disorders: The Journal of Treatment and Prevention*; vice president of the Eating Disorders Coalition for Research, Policy, and Action; a Founding Member and Fellow of the Academy for Eating Disorders; a Founder of the National Eating Disorders Association; and the 2007 recipient of its Lori Irving Award for Excellence in Eating Disorders Awareness and Prevention.

All suffering is bearable
if it is seen as part of a story.
ISAK DINESEN

In an interview on National Public Radio, Augusten Burroughs said that "perfect" lives don't make good stories. He felt compelled to write as a salve for his pain. If not for the struggle that called for expression, he said that writing would have been far too much work. I understand.

I was inspired to write *Riptide: Struggling with and Resurfacing from a Daughter's Eating Disorder* while my oldest daughter, Erin, was in the throes of an ultimately fatal eating disorder. As a parent who is also a therapist, I was plagued by my inability to even slow her worsening condition over a 10-year period. This experience challenged my sense of control over my life, my identity as a competent and compassionate person, and the values by which I lived and defined myself. I questioned my merit, whether life was worth living, and how I as a mother could survive the life-and-death battle that was being played out in my daughter's psyche and body. As a committed therapist whose daily work is helping others heal and grow, I felt intense shame and self-consciousness about not being able to save my own child. I now understand that many parents of eating-disordered, mentally ill, and/or chemically dependent children feel that shame.

As someone once said, pain is inevitable, but suffering is optional. I wrote *Riptide* to offer hope, inspiration, reassurance, and practical guidance for families with a child dealing with an eating disorder, addiction, and/or mental illness. In addition, professionals who work with these families will gain deeper understanding of these parents' guilt, self-doubt, and destructive self-sacrifice.

Riptide is the story of my relationship with my daughter throughout her disease. Like a set of Russian nesting dolls, the story of my struggle with Erin occurred within the context of my story of myself, which was shaped by the family legacy I inherited. How I saw myself as a woman and how I related to food and my body were powerful influences on Erin's development. My marriage to Erin's father was part of that picture, and our divorce disrupted the stability she needed at a crucial point in her development.

And then there was the genetic tendency toward mental illness, of which we were unaware at the time, as well as the neurological impact of the rheumatic fever Erin contracted when she was nine years old. All of these factors complicated the quest for understanding that became a maze with more walls than exits.

As the years passed, I learned that the only real exit from that maze was keeping my heart open and having compassion for myself, no matter what happened. I slowly learned that being with my daughter in a loving way and grieving and letting go were essential to maintaining my sanity as hers gave way to the disease. I regressed often during this process that took years.

Despite my loving, supportive second husband and wise friends, I often felt alone — unaware of how similar my struggles were to those of other parents. Since then, I've learned that many others are asking the same questions I asked. As author and workshop leader Sam Keen wisely stated, "The questions we ask determine the answers we get."

This book is more about identifying the questions we are asking ourselves, reframing them when they are intrinsically dead-end and destructive, and learning how to honor ourselves as we love and support our children through their struggles. When am I helpful? When am I refusing to acknowledge my helplessness? How do I manage my own emotions, especially fear, anger, and grief, so that I can make decisions with which I can live? Where does my responsibility end and my child's begin? How do I reconcile my unconditional love with setting limits that my child may experience as hurtful or uncaring? These are some of the questions I asked myself, and it took years for me to overcome the undertow of guilt that belied the smooth surface of my calm control.

In recounting my experiences, I changed most of the names of the individuals involved and did my best to recall and record happenings, conversations, and my thoughts at the time as accurately as possible. However, my purpose is not to provide a history, but to tell a story based on actual events. In dreams and fables, myths and parables, the literal events are there to carry meaning. Similarly with *Riptide*, what actually happened is less important than what I told myself at the time. How those interpretations evolved as I healed and grew through deep reflection has enabled me to move on with my life.

Spiritual leader and writer Ernest Holmes advised, "Refuse to carry the corpse of a mistaken yesterday." For years my heart was weighted with regret over the times that weariness, frustration, and hurt — rather than steady, soft-hearted compassion — ruled my choices. My grieving was hobbled by guilt for not having always been the best version of myself. It's been much easier for me to make room for the imperfections of others than for mine — to encourage my clients, family, and friends to bury their corpses, even as I continued to carry my own.

My hope is that relating my experience will provide you with the comfort that you aren't alone — especially in any feelings of helplessness and shame — and support you in finding your own internal rudder when confronted with these inevitable questions. The 13th-century poet Rumi wrote, "Beyond ideas of rightdoing and wrongdoing there is a field. I'll meet you there." This is the field in which my story stands. This is the field of the soft and open heart. As Buddhist teacher and writer Stephen Levine said, "We can't make room for someone else's pain until we make room for our own." This book is about making room for the pain that is inevitable when your child is troubled.

The Mother Knot

The challenge was not to do
the impossible – but to learn
to live with the possible.

SUE BENDER

As I opened the door of Erin's apartment on a bright summer afternoon in 1999, I took a deep breath. My 22-year-old daughter lay on the daybed in her living room, bird-like legs stretched out over rumpled sheets. She was propped up on one elbow, drawing in a sketch pad, and her ankles were wrapped in thick white gauze and bandages. I tried not to grimace.

I was used to scanning my daughter's body for signs of deterioration, though it seemed impossible to imagine her more emaciated than she was. Functional starvation, if there was such a term, best described her condition. And now the meager flesh that remained on her ankles had been scalded a week ago when she'd dropped a pot of boiling water on the floor — undoubtedly because her arms no longer had the strength to lift it off the stove. I hadn't realized it was quite this bad.

Erin looked up at me. "They're just not healing as fast as they should," she said, her tone resigned.

I glimpsed the edge of a raw open wound on one spindly leg. Erin was five feet tall and weighed about 60 pounds. How could her starving little body sustain the shock of these deep burns, much less keep her alive? Were painkillers at least softening the agony?

The burns were bad, but I could handle that. Injuries heal. It was the rest of her that, over the past decade of brutal anorexia and depression, left me limp. I felt as though I'd washed up on the beach after alternately struggling to pull my daughter to shore and trying to free myself from a stranglehold that threatened to pull me under along with her.

Close friends knew our family's private pain, but the community at large could only guess at what was wrong when they saw Erin walk up Main Street, her skeletal frame somewhat disguised by baggy clothes, each step an obvious effort. She was a familiar sight in town. Weighed down by her ever-present tote bag stuffed with artificial sweetener packets, herbal tea, sketch pad and colored pencils, she would stop in at the espresso shop and ask for hot water for her tea, or perhaps meet an unemployed friend at Mister Donut. She identified with those whose lives were on the periphery of the 9-to-5 world. Once a gifted student, dancer, and artist, Erin now qualified for Social Security Disability benefits. Instead of anticipating graduate school or a challenging job, she hoped for an apartment in the housing program for the disabled, and underwent partial hospitalization three days a week.

We had exiled Erin to this small apartment several months after she returned from her final failed long-term treatment. She was 21, and after years of having her alternating every few months between living with her father and with me, it was intolerable for either of us to have her in our home. The chronic stealing, bingeing, and purging that ruled her life made living with her a nightmare of missing money, discarded food containers, and clogged drains. Holiday celebrations and family birthday dinners were strained by our tense, surreptitious monitoring. Would the festive meal be flushed down the toilet once again, after she'd filled her shrunken stomach with turkey, mashed potatoes, and homemade rolls? Or would we feel equally frustrated and powerless as her bony jaw chewed, trance-like, on unadorned salad and naked vegetables? She either gorged or fasted, and we'd long since learned that there was nothing we could do. The happiness and well-being of my three younger daughters helped to redeem my motherhood and cushion my despair. Yet I was Erin's mother, too, and I feared I had failed her.

I walked across the room and sat down on the daybed, the weight of my body pulling her closer to me. Gently, I stroked her head.

"I've thought of so many ways to commit suicide," she said flatly. "But each one I've either already tried, or known someone where it didn't work or was even worse afterwards. I'm not going to try anymore."

I flashed back to the night she'd swallowed half a bottle of pills. Why was she telling me this now? Did she think I would be relieved, or did she want me to know how desperate she still felt? I didn't say anything. All my words had been used up, my heart frayed by the fear, sadness, and frustration that had consumed me for a decade. I continued to stroke her hair. That I could do.

The nearby university's carillon bells rang twice, reminding me that I had to be home in an hour to start seeing afternoon clients. "What can I get for you?" I asked.

She ticked off her list of safe foods: "Cabbage, frozen spinach, and tuna in water."

I assumed she had hidden away her stash of pretzels, animal crackers, and popcorn — favorite binge foods — or else was too embarrassed to ask me to buy those, too.

"Are you sure that's all?" I questioned.

She nodded, and I leaned over to kiss the top of her head before I left. Even her scalp felt thin.

I didn't notice the knot in my stomach until I was in the car. Driving to the store, I kept replaying the image of Erin's injured limbs and large, pleading eyes. The eyes of a prisoner. Several minutes later I pulled into an empty space in front of the grocery store, turned off the ignition, and took my brain off auto-pilot. I welcomed the cool air and familiar smell as I stepped into the store, the knot in my stomach loosening with the illusion of normalcy. I'm just picking up some food for my daughter. What could be easier than that?

But nothing with her was easy anymore. Not shopping for her meager rations, not washing her child-size clothes. Not understanding how to be the parent of a child who was disappearing day by day. My fierce, protective mother-love battled with weary despair, anger at the betrayal of my dreams for her, and the tormenting fear that it was somehow my fault, after all. What did it mean that my heart ached with love, yet I wanted to run at the sight of her? I didn't know what was real or true anymore. "Father Knows Best" had given way to "Mother Knows Nothing."

I drove back to her apartment with the white plastic sack of rations. As I put spinach and cabbage into the refrigerator, Erin looked up from watching a soap opera.

"Thanks, Mom."

I kissed her on the top of her head and left, the screen door clanging shut behind me.

In 1989, when she was 12, Erin made a pact with the devil, a disease called anorexia. Years of therapy and multiple hospitalizations did little to loosen the grip of her eating-disordered mind, and she battled and colluded with that demon through most of her teenage years and into her early twenties. I felt trapped in a nightmare that made no sense, and I didn't know how to wake up. I didn't know it was possible to wake up. I wept and ranted my feelings in my morning journal, finally facing, after nearly a decade of fear, frustration, and sadness, the inescapable reality that a beautiful woman would never emerge from the stunted, skeletal body my daughter now had.

As Erin's struggle with anorexia and bulimia consumed her life and nearly devoured mine, I lived in parallel universes — the waking world in which I functioned with apparent ease and confidence, and the invisible nightmare world of fading hope, helplessness, and even suicidal desperation. Only a handful of people knew the surreal ordeal that shadowed my daily life. At times I felt that she and I were in mortal combat, and only one of us would win. She was killing me slowly with her self-destruction and her need for me to save her. I felt like I would be the one to die if I couldn't make her surrender.

I surprised myself with my demonic craziness. It clawed at my heart and refused to relinquish its grip on my rational mind. I waged my war silently, in the quiet of my early morning journal writing. Meanwhile, I honed my skills as a psychotherapist, built my career, and, with my second husband, blended our family of five children — his son and my four daughters. We spent countless evenings in the gym, playing volleyball and basketball games, celebrating our other children's rites of passage. That normalcy was the tip of my emotional iceberg, while the mass of my fear, helplessness, and grief lay hidden to those who only skimmed the surface of our lives.

We seemed to go on as if all was well, but I ached for the child who taught her younger sisters and neighborhood playmates to dance and do cartwheels in the yard, and whose infectious giggle sparkled in the air when we watched *The Muppet Show* or *Fraggle Rock*. She had the broad shoulders and narrow hips of a competitive swimmer and the lithe, muscled legs of a ballerina. In early photos from those happier times, her large green eyes look wistful, as if she knew her loveliness would be short-lived.

As a psychotherapist, the motto "Physician, heal thyself" only added to my guilt and frustration. What kind of mother would change the locks on her house to keep out her own daughter, especially when that daughter is a tiny, frail wraith who can barely carry her own weight? What kind of mother could take the rest of the family on vacation and leave one of her offspring behind in a dingy little apartment? At the time, those decisions seemed to be the only options for keeping Erin's behaviors from eclipsing any joy and ease in our family life. Nonetheless, the judgment I visited upon myself and imagined from others rang in my ears, often drowning out the quiet voice that said, "It's okay for you to live your life and be happy."

Happy Days

You, too, have come into the
world to do this, to go easy, to be
filled with light, and to shine.

MARY OLIVER

On October 5, 1976, sunshine streamed into the hospital room where I sat holding Erin Leah, my firstborn, to my breast. I smiled, filled with postpartum relief and peace, as her little mouth gently and determinedly sucked nourishment from my body. The realization that I was a mother and that this was my child was still sinking in since her birth the evening before. I suddenly knew that we were meant to be together, and I would do everything possible to provide her with the best life I could.

In the wake of how Erin's life unfolded, which I would have been horrified to imagine that day, I find reassurance and comfort in Kahlil Gibran's words from *The Prophet*:

Your children are not your children.

They are the sons and daughters of Life's longing for itself.

They come through you but not from you,

And though they are with you yet they belong not to you.

You may give them your love but not your thoughts,

For they have their own thoughts.

You may house their bodies but not their souls,

For their souls dwell in the house of to-morrow, which you cannot visit,

not even in your dreams.

You may strive to be like them, but seek not to make them like you.

For life goes not backward nor tarries with yesterday.

And so I choose to believe that she came to me and through me for reasons of her own, and I am grateful that I was blessed with her for the time we had together.

Psychologists hypothesize that our memory of painful events is far keener and more powerful than our ability to recall happy and benign times — the way a car accident overshadows an uneventful vacation. It's thought to be a survival strategy; the acute memory of painful past experiences makes us better prepared for future dangers. Because Erin's life was such a struggle, the painful memories eclipsed the happy times. Recently I went through the many smiling photos from her childhood before the disorder and my heart lightened. I felt the shining essence of who she was visible from where it had been hidden for so long by the moon shadow of her disorder, and I could remember and honor the delightful, energetic, bright, and creative child she had been for so long.

In 1977, when Erin was eight months old, my husband Roger and I moved from Albany to Bemidji, Minnesota, for his first college teaching position. The distance from our families in upstate New York was difficult, but I adjusted quickly to the small-town life by making friends with other young mothers. I reveled in the domestic rhythms and routines of my days. Erin was a happy toddler, always actively exploring, and I was delighted to learn I was pregnant again when she was 18 months old.

Several months later, I started transitioning Erin to a bed so the new baby could have her crib. One afternoon I tucked her into her new bed for a nap and went downstairs to catch up on household chores. When I peeked into her bedroom an hour later, I found her fast asleep in the nest she'd made with her blanket in the little wooden chest a friend had made when she was born — an early, playful metaphor for a life in which she was determined to make her own bed and lie in it.

Although she slept well at night, she fell into the habit of waking up around 1 a.m. and calling for a bottle of water. I worried that once the new baby was born, I wouldn't have the energy for any additional nighttime demands, but I didn't want Erin crying herself back to sleep, either. One evening as we sat in her brightly wallpapered room reading the *Best Word Book Ever!* (Others may experience divine intervention through praying to a favorite saint or the Blessed Virgin, but mine came through Richard Scarry.) She turned to the airplane page.

"Honey, you know how Grandma comes here to visit and then goes back home on an airplane?"

She nodded, wide-eyed. She had a special bond with Roger's mother, Carol, who would visit for several weeks at a time.

I continued, "Well, bottle went bye-bye on the airplane, just like Grandma."

We read a few more pages, and I tucked her in, not knowing if the seed I had planted in her fertile imagination would sprout. During the middle of the night I woke up to her little voice softly chanting, "Bottle, bye-bye . . . bottle, bye-bye." And she never asked for a bottle again. Years later when I remembered her soft voice in the night, I would long for such painless solutions.

Despite Roger's occasional bouts of temper, our family life had a pleasant domestic rhythm. Roger's academic schedule allowed summers at home, which gave us the opportunity to take day trips and explore the many small lakes in the area. One hot August day when Carol was visiting, we all went to the beach at Lake Benjamin, a short drive from Bemidji. Carol was pushing my second daughter, Jenna, in her stroller at the edge of the sand, by the woods, as Roger and I played in the water with Erin. "I want to give your mother a break," I told him after I'd cooled off in the water, and I headed for the beach. I assumed he'd heard me, but he didn't, and he began swimming on his own, assuming I was with Erin. When I reached Carol and the baby, I looked back out at the water and panicked. I didn't see Erin's wavy blond head anywhere. "Where's Erin?" I screamed to Roger. He swung around and dove underwater. After a few long seconds he was holding Erin up above the surface and carried her to where I was standing on the beach. My heart was still pounding with the possibility that we might have lost her as I ran to hold her wet little body close. She wasn't choking or gagging, so I knew she couldn't have been under too long. The only one of us unshaken was Erin, who said, "Mommy put her face on Daddy and pulled me out of the water."

Later that day after the girls were tucked in for the night, Carol brought up the near tragedy and Erin's words. "I think what she saw was the face of our Blessed Mother." Carol believed there had been a divine intervention. Though at times I dismissed Carol's spiritual interpretations of mundane situations — seeing the name on a passing truck as a message from God or particular cloud formations symbolizing guardian angels — I had no other way of explaining what Erin had seen and said.

From the time Erin was a toddler, just learning to make marks with crayons, her drawing seemed inspired by another dimension. I had just come downstairs from changing Jenna's diaper one afternoon, and saw Erin kneeling in front of the coffee table with Carol beside her on the couch. Erin was drawing stick figures with large circles on each side of their triangular bases. "What are you drawing, Honey?" Carol asked. "Those are wheel angels, Grandma," Erin replied matter-of-factly. I chalked her response up to a child's imagination, but Carol insisted that there was a category of angels called "wheel angels" that she had recently learned about in her study of mystical beings. Though Erin's drawings became more skillfully detailed over the years, they were seldom representational. She was absorbed for hours creating colorful designs and elaborately detailed scenes of whimsical creatures — it seemed as if she drew inspiration from a transcendent realm.

Erin was also an active explorer of her physical world. Some of her escapades landed us in the ER, but many were simply harmless little adventures. Several months after Jenna was born, I awoke after midnight to her crying. More than 10 pounds at birth, Jenna nursed every two hours, day or night, for months. After nursing Jenna and laying her back in her crib, I noticed a dim light coming from downstairs. Misty, our Australian sheepdog, would have barked if there had been an intruder, I told myself, so I didn't feel the need to awaken Roger. I followed the light down the stairs and through the dark living room to the open basement door. As soon as I got to the top of the steps, I saw Erin in her turquoise footed sleeper sitting in the middle of the cat box at the base of the steps with the litter scoop in her hand. I laughed as I ran down the steps, saying, "It's not a sandbox, Honey!" After washing her off in the bathtub and putting her in a clean sleeper, she quickly fell asleep. If there were other middle-of-the-night escapades, I slept through them.

Though Roger and I enjoyed our life in Bemidji, we missed our families. Ariel was born when Jenna was only 21 months old, and with each new baby, the longing to be closer to our families grew stronger. I wanted my mother to be part of her granddaughters' lives without having to drive halfway across the country to see each other, and though Carol flew out to be with us several times a year, it wasn't the same as being within driving distance. We were delighted when Roger was hired for a position in a small state university in rural north central Pennsylvania. On a rainy day in late June 1981, we loaded all our furniture and belongings in a U-Haul truck and trailer. I followed Roger in our family station wagon with Carol and our three young daughters, now four years, two years, and eight months old. Roger had the cat and dog in the truck cab with him.

Dance recitals were a major community event in our new town, with the auditorium at the university filled to capacity with families and friends. At her first recital, five-year-old Erin was excited to perform. As instructed, I had sewn pastel Velcro circles onto her maroon leotard and pinned a red one onto her hair. She and 20 other "polka dots" kicked their chubby little legs and spun in all directions, the audience howling with laughter. Those pre-schoolers were trying so hard to get it right, and no one cared if they did. Afterward, when we went out for ice cream, she announced, "I can't wait to do that again!" Unlike her self-conscious mother, she delighted in the opportunity to perform, and, by the time she was 10, she was performing acrobatic solos at the recitals, grinning the whole time.

In one of my favorite photos, Erin is looking up at the camera with a wide smile as she buckles the sandal on her left foot. She's wearing a black leotard and black tights with a short, flouncy, red calico skirt — her dance recital costume the year she was nine. In the recital photo from the following year, she sits in a perfect split, her arms gracefully extended. She relished being on stage. When I was young, on the other hand, I was sick to my stomach before piano recitals. When I was 15 I played a Beethoven sonata and left the stage without a single memory of having done so.

For Erin, there were no pre-performance jitters. It was pure joy. In the summer she would gather her sisters and neighborhood playmates, and with a favorite song on the boom box, she tried to teach them how to dance. She had a natural grace I could only dream of, and it seemed to me there was nothing at which she couldn't excel. She was only 10 when Roger took her down to the town park to perform a dance she had choreographed for a talent contest at the Fourth of July festivities. Though the Annie Lennox tape got stuck a few times, Erin kept her cool and won the contest.

Ever determined and full of energy, she was only six years old when the Episcopal Church that Roger and I attended with the girls sponsored a bike-a-thon to benefit St. Jude's Children's Hospital. All the children were encouraged to get sponsors for a dollar a mile. Erin collected a number of sponsors from our neighbors and relatives. As the children rode their bicycles around the university track, their laps were counted. That Sunday in church, the coordinator of the bike-a-thon announced that of all the participants, Erin, the youngest, had ridden the farthest — seven miles — and that she looked like she would have kept going if they hadn't run out of time. Like *The Little Engine That Could* that we read together at bedtime, my little girl, once she'd made up her mind, wasn't going to give up.

3

Falling Down the Rabbit Hole

What are you supposed to do,
when what is happening can't be,
and the old rules no longer apply?

ANNE LAMOTT

I was chopping onions and grating cheese for our dinner quiche on a warm September afternoon when Erin was in seventh grade, and I noticed her focusing intently on something she was writing in a spiral notebook.

"What are you working on, honey?" I asked.

"We're supposed to write down everything we eat for Life Skills," she replied.

I left the cutting board to look over her shoulder. Breakfast: one half-cup oatmeal; Lunch: six carrot sticks, two slices of turkey, apple. That was it. No sandwich. No cookies or chips. Hardly enough for an active 13-year-old to eat and be fueled for the day.

She'll eat a hearty supper, I told myself. *Quiche is a favorite. Always a perfectionist, she's just taking this assignment too seriously. After all, it's only seventh grade homework, and she's been moody lately. What adolescent isn't?*

Several weeks later, as I walked onto the front porch of our remodeled old farm house, I bristled at the sound of Jane Fonda's voice blaring from the television in the living room: "Kick, kick, three, four. . . ." It was the end of another emotionally draining day in the early months of my new job, and I longed for my blue jeans, a baggy T-shirt, and the comforting routine of preparing dinner. I rarely knew if my counseling with distressed families had any lasting or even immediate impact, so shedding my work clothes and fixing a meal was a welcome respite and provided a predictable outcome for my effort.

Instead of relief, I faced Erin jumping and leg-lifting to my old workout video. Last year's pale blue dance leotard sagged on her lean torso and gaped at the top of her shrinking thighs. Her chest was flat where budding breasts had emerged several months before. That school assignment meant to promote healthy awareness had backfired as her mind latched onto tallying calories like a penny-pinching Scrooge.

"Hi, honey!" I said brightly, as I dodged her swinging arms and legs to make my way to the kitchen.

Though I bristled at seeing her burn off calories she wasn't consuming, I didn't show it. I knew by now that would only backfire — she would exercise even harder or run upstairs and refuse to come down for dinner. Unending piles of laundry to wash and meals to prepare had been easy compared to this.

Later that evening as we sat down for dinner, I winced at the sight of her plate — a mound of unadorned green beans and a small slice of chicken breast.

"Don't you want some potatoes?" I gingerly suggested, "or a slice of French bread?"

"I'm fine! I'm not hungry!" she snapped.

I plowed ahead as if I weren't walking onto a field of land-mines.

"Honey, I'm worried about you. You hardly had anything for lunch, and now you're not eating enough to keep a bird alive."

"Leave me alone!" she cried, throwing back her chair, running up the stairs, and slamming her bedroom door.

My heart hammered against my chest, and I pushed my plate to the side. Paralyzed by frustration, I wondered, *What do I do now?* Where was the line between being weak and giving her space? Between being a strong parent and a tyrant?

As I cleared the table and loaded the dishwasher, I decided to call the next morning to make an appointment with our family doctor.

"It's just a routine physical," I told Erin.

A few days later, after Erin stepped off the scale in the examining room, the doctor looked at me with alarm: "She's lost 11 pounds. We're looking at anorexia."

Feeling a mix of dread and relief, I thought, *There is a problem. I have the right to be upset.*

The doctor handed me a business card. The bold blue lettering read, "Nutrition Clinic," and I wondered why I'd never heard of it.

"Make an appointment and see what they suggest," she continued. "They can do a thorough assessment and come up with a plan to help her get healthy again."

Erin was quiet, looking down at the floor, her jaw clenched. Round One was over. We were back in our respective corners. I had no idea how she would react to Round Two, but at least there was a next step I could take.

My divorce from Roger had been finalized several months earlier. We had agreed that I would stay in the house with primary custody of our four girls. He had bought land and built a small home several miles outside of town. Despite some lingering resentment, we worked well with each other when it came to our daughters. Through the three previous years of graduate school and clinical internships I was able to adjust my schedule to their school hours. Once I was hired as a clinical social worker in a sexual abuse treatment program 30 miles away, I didn't get home until 6 p.m., and I had to count on Roger to pick them up from school and supervise Ariel and Jocelyn, the younger two, until I arrived. I had always been available to pick up my children from school, to take them home in the middle of the day if they were ill, or to drop off a forgotten lunch, but now I was too far away to come running on short notice.

Besides the adjustment to working full time with the added commute, I agonized about what was happening in the families I counseled and my ability to make a difference. I've never forgotten the seven-year-old girl who was afraid to tell a caseworker she was sexually abused at night by her father. No one could guarantee her safety. She had a roof over her head and food, so as long as she was too afraid to reveal her nightly ordeal to the caseworker, the Department of Social Services said their hands, like hers, were tied.

This was the kind of situation that broke my heart — such a contrast to my benign upbringing and the cozy nest I'd provided for my four daughters. Despite our divorce, their lives looked secure and well-padded compared with those nightmare scenarios I heard firsthand every day. How could a child of mine be anything but fine?

When I drove Erin to her first appointment at the clinic, I chatted about our plans for next summer's vacation, hoping to distract her from dwelling on what might be ahead. But she was quiet in the passenger seat beside me, staring straight ahead.

Maybe she's just nervous, I told myself.

Not being one of those people who can talk to a lamppost, I gave up on trying to engage my mute daughter. After 40 minutes of icy silence, I pulled into the circular drive in front of the large, white Victorian that housed the clinic and parked the old Toyota. Erin wordlessly followed me through the front foyer into the bright, homey waiting room, with its high ceilings and tall windows. Carolyn Hodges, the founder and director, welcomed us with an open smile. Though she was younger than I had expected, she exuded both warmth and competence, and I liked her immediately.

After I filled out all the paperwork, she ushered Erin through a series of tests to assess her body's current metabolism and percentages of lean and fat weight. An hour later, Carolyn called us into a small office to go over the results.

"Her weight doesn't tell the whole story," she explained, "which is why we do the body composition testing and metabolic check. Erin's body is already stripping muscle tissue because she's been restricting so much."

She turned to Erin as she continued to educate us about how the body, in its attempt to protect itself from starvation, holds onto fat and burns up muscle tissue instead.

"It's a survival strategy that has evolved to keep the species alive during times when food is scarce," she said. "Even though you lose weight and keep getting smaller, you're losing muscle and storing more fat."

As she spoke, I watched Erin's face, hoping for a flicker of interest or concern. It was blank. I knew she understood everything Carolyn said, but did it matter? I couldn't tell. Carolyn handed Erin a list of foods she could choose from for each meal, to make sure that she had an adequate balance of protein and carbohydrates to start restoring her body to a healthy lean-to-fat ratio. Erin glanced at the list, still expressionless.

"When should we come back?" I asked, looking at Carolyn with relief and gratitude.

"Have Brandi set up an appointment next week, and I want Erin to see the doctor then, too," Carolyn answered with a smile.

Erin folded the list and stood up. *At least she's not arguing, and she doesn't look too mad*, I thought.

"Come on, honey," I said. "Let's stop at the store and see if there's anything we need for you."

I put my arm around her shoulders, and we walked over to the reception desk to schedule the next appointment.

Roger and I took turns driving Erin to the Nutrition Clinic 30 miles away and to her therapy appointments, which also included us at times. I assumed that it was only a matter of time before she was "cured." After all, this wasn't cancer or some other deadly illness. She had excelled at everything — gymnastics, dance, drawing, and academics — there was no other possible future in my mind. I had to believe that my achievement-motivated daughter would conquer this problem too. I didn't realize that for her, anorexia *was* an achievement.

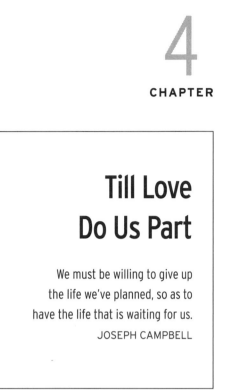

Till Love Do Us Part

We must be willing to give up
the life we've planned, so as to
have the life that is waiting for us.

JOSEPH CAMPBELL

In the summer of 1969, I participated in a seven-week study tour to Germany sponsored by the State University of New York at Albany, where I was enrolled to start college in the fall. Several weeks into the trip, as I was reading on a park bench in the small Bavarian town where we were studying, one of the young men on the tour sat down beside me. He was tall, attractive, with dark wavy hair and blue-gray eyes. I was surprised to have him notice me. He asked about the novel I was reading and spoke of his enthusiasm for Ayn Rand. He said his name was Roger.

Throughout the remainder of the trip, I spent a lot of time with him. On our last night in Germany, as he walked me back to my room, he gave me his chunky silver identification bracelet, and — I'm loathe to admit — my first kiss. I lay in bed that night embarrassed, disappointed, and relieved it had finally happened.

That September, after my parents had helped me move into my dormitory room and were back on the highway headed toward Buffalo, I wandered over to the Rathskeller Student Union. Roger had just walked in, and I told myself that our perfect timing was a good omen. From then on we ate most of our meals together, went to the Rathskeller on Saturday nights for beer and pretzels, and enjoyed discussing politics, religion, and philosophy. Roger became a haven from having to challenge the social anxiety I'd hoped to leave behind in high school.

I thought we were perfect. Within months we were the center of one another's little universe. The spring of our freshman year, on the morning after Roger asked me to marry him, I floated to my classes, oblivious to my surroundings and buoyed by the relief of belonging and being wanted. All my twinges of discomfort vanished at the prospect of being saved — I would be normal and have a family. I loved him for loving me.

On our wedding day in May 1971, when I was 19 years old, I allowed no room for doubt. It was the happiest day of my life. I had no last-minute pangs. No impulses to run. I was convinced we were perfect for each other. Doubts would mean I hadn't thought it out well enough, which would mean I might be doing something wrong.

For 17 years I acted the part of the perfect wife and mother, secure in the knowledge that I had proven my worth. Who could doubt this picture? We looked happy. We acted happy. Because we never fought, we thought we were happy.

Roger had spent years studying Native American and Eastern spirituality, and we had a circle of friends who gathered weekly to talk and silently meditate. Though I was an active participant in our group, my daily energy was consumed with our children and household. I resented it when he said he was doing me a favor if he watched the girls while I went out for a run. I tiptoed around him when he withdrew into irritable silence, never knowing what might send him into a rage. As frustrated as I can now admit I was by the unacknowledged walls around our feelings and Roger's unwillingness to take on more than a minimal share of the parenting, he must have been disappointed, too. I was a reluctant moon to his sun, and for all my efficient housekeeping and attentive parenting, I never reached for him. Our marriage was a well-oiled machine without any soul.

In March 1984, Roger returned from a weekend workshop on spiritual dance given by a Native American medicine woman. I stayed home to care for our girls, then ages two, four, six, and eight. When the van pulled into our driveway on Sunday evening, I went out to greet them. Roger was holding onto our friend Celia's arm as he stepped down like an unsteady 80-year-old. He looked shaken and said he felt as though he'd been broken in two by an invisible force during the trip back. Celia had cradled him for hours as he trembled and wept.

"I feel like I have to learn to walk again," he said, once we were together inside the house. "I've been seeing past lives and the earth doesn't feel solid — it's like I'm falling through it."

After this experience Roger was, for a while, a softer, gentler version of himself, gushing with love and gratitude for me, the children, and everyone we knew. He was more patient and playful with the girls and even apologized if he snapped because his nerves were so exposed and raw.

One night a few months later when Roger was earthbound again, I was sitting on the living room couch, legs tucked under me, flipping through the pages of the latest *Redbook* magazine when Roger came into the room.

"I need to tell you something," he said, sitting down beside me. I looked up at him, surprised by his somber tone and serious expression.

"I've fallen in love with Celia."

I was too stunned to reply.

"We have a spiritual connection. . . ."

What else he may have said I didn't hear. Without thinking I detoured around the temptation to indulge my rage and, looking into his frightened eyes, I said, "Do what you need to do." Those words came from a place I didn't know existed.

It was late by then, nearly 10 p.m., but sleep wasn't an option. I headed out the front door. The sky was studded with stars and the neighborhood was quiet, except for the sound of an occasional car on another block. I focused on the trees in black profile against an even blacker sky and headed up the hill next to our house, willing the quiet, familiar scenery to swaddle my thrashing insides, my jangled mind careening against the neat, white walls of my expected life like a racquetball. I walked until midnight, hoping to get tired enough to succumb to slumber. After a hot shower, I crawled into bed next to Roger. He reached for me, but I rolled toward the edge of the mattress. Letting him hold me now, or have more of me, would feel like conciliation, and I wasn't ready for that. I wanted him to hurt — to be worried about what I might say, do, and feel.

Later, when I looked back on the spontaneous choice I'd made to, in essence, give him permission to have an affair, I didn't regret it. Even though I could have strong-armed him into ending it with Celia, I knew that would not have solved anything. He told me he still loved me, and I believed him. Celia wasn't a replacement for me. She could be to him what I had never been and would never be. And he wasn't ready to mess up his life that much.

My acceptance never turned to complacency, however. Anxiety coursed through my body. The marriage I'd believed in was a mirage. Night after night, though I fell asleep exhausted, I awoke at midnight, wide awake, my mind racing. When I tried to eat, my stomach was in knots after a few bites. Even though there was no imminent disruption to my life, nothing was the same. I was falling through cracks I'd never noticed. Faith in my ever-competent control was a fantasy. Who was that staring back from the shattered mirror of my life?

I had wondered about the smallish, wiry man I noticed at times who always seemed to be rushing somewhere, his head in front of his body. I assumed he taught at the college, probably in the art department or theater, with his Beethoven hair and intense focus. Yet there he was in the doorway of his piano studio, the embodied voice with whom I'd spoken over the telephone to arrange Erin's first piano lesson. He greeted Erin and me with a warm smile on that hot July day, nearly three years before Roger's announcement. Erin was almost six, and I was eight months pregnant with Jocelyn.

Once Jocelyn was born, Andrew agreed to teach Erin at our home to make it easier for me. After the lessons were over, he and I would chat about books and music we both enjoyed. Roger liked Andrew as well, and soon we were socializing with Andrew and his wife, Karen. They had married five years earlier, squeezing her five children and his two-year-old son, Zane, into a small ranch house at the south end of town. Two-and-a-half years later, after the strain of their large blended family and a hand-to-mouth economy had taken its toll on their marriage, Karen moved out. Both she and Andrew seemed relieved as their divorce proceeded quickly, with no resistance and little to divide.

Meanwhile, my marriage looked unchanged to those on the outside. I didn't want to talk about it at my peer counseling group because several of Roger's colleagues' wives were members. The one venue that was meant to provide me with a place to clear out troubling feelings was out of bounds because of the tabloid nature of news in such a small town. Strangely, I wasn't angry with Celia. She had been a friend through our church, I liked her, and I knew she felt terrible that I had been hurt. I agreed to keep her relationship with Roger secret. As a result, there were few friends with whom I could speak freely.

But Andrew was one. Roger encouraged me to spend time with him, and it wasn't long before Andrew was my primary confidant. I was at ease with him whether we were bantering playfully or discussing how to deal with our serious life changes. I wanted him to want me, though I had no idea what I would do if he did. I was still a married woman and hadn't allowed even the thought of another man to enter my mind for 15 years. But whenever I saw Andrew, everything and everyone else became a backdrop. All those corny clichés about leaping and melting hearts felt real and profound, and I could have been a country music poster girl.

Soon I wanted more than a fraternal goodnight hug. One evening as we sat facing each other on opposite ends of his couch I began to massage his feet, willing him to feel the love and desire pouring through my fingers. My practical, planning mind was off-line, and I felt a passion I'd never known. Since the rules in my marriage had been broken, anything was possible.

He looked up with his clear blue eyes and said, "I think we're falling in love."

In 1986, I began a three-year master's degree program in social work. At that point the girls ranged in age from four to 10, so I did my class work during the few hours when school and pre-school overlapped. There could be no changes for a while, not only because I couldn't support myself, but because even the thought of divorce roused instant panic in me. Though Roger knew I was in love with Andrew, he wanted to keep our marriage intact, as if we could indefinitely have our relationships on the side like condiments to an otherwise bland main dish. He spent what time he could with Celia, and I saw or spoke with Andrew daily.

But Andrew wasn't willing to stay on the sidelines of my life. I knew it wasn't fair to him, and I was chafing at living a lie. Even though we were all open with each other, what my life appeared to be in the community was not what it was. I didn't want to go on like that either, but I was afraid to confront Roger, to upset, disrupt, and possibly damage the girls, and to give up the financial security that marriage to Roger assured.

In contrast, Andrew's lifestyle challenged all the predictability and security I had believed were the hallmarks of responsibility and success. I had always been a straight line kind of person, rarely taking a side trip to explore the scenery, but Andrew's life was a saga of detours. After a lifetime of adventure that included a stint in a seminary, working as a cab driver, and joining the Peace Corps, Andrew was now cobbling together a living teaching piano, working at a facility for developmentally disabled women, and using a student loan to complete his degree in music therapy. How could I leave the perfect family, steady income, and retirement plan for a 43-year-old man who had lived in a treehouse with a woodstove, bed, and grand piano (a living arrangement abandoned when he gained custody of his two-year-old son, Zane), and who thought a 401k was the airplane that preceded the 747? I had four daughters to think about.

During the summer of 1986, when Roger and I were uncertain about the future of our relationship, we visited my sister Brenda and her husband Dave at Dave's parents' large log home on Smith Mountain Lake. Erin was 10 years old when she and her sisters stood along the deck railing, smiling at the camera after an active afternoon of swimming.

The following summer, when I was wrestling with whether or not to divorce Roger and about to enter my second year of graduate school, I took advantage of an invitation once again from Brenda's in-laws to bring the girls and stay with them in Fredericksburg, Virginia, for a few days while Brenda, Dave, and their baby daughter Sonja were back east again from where they lived in Arizona. The lasting image from that trip is the photo of Dave acting as group leader as the girls, oldest to youngest, strode behind him along the cement wall of the large rectangular pool in the National Mall.

During our touring that day, I learned that a Gauguin Exhibit was at the National Gallery. Erin and I both wanted to go, so later that afternoon, Brenda and Dave took the younger girls back to his parents' and Erin and I shared the thrill of seeing and being transported by the vibrant energy of Paul Gauguin's paintings. I was inspired by the bright, bold beauty of his work and the daring of his decision to scrap convention and move to Tahiti to pursue his passion. Perhaps it was more than the power of his art that had me feeling high for several days after that.

Once home, I had to wrestle again with the questions at the heart of my marital quandary. What was real? What really mattered? What did I have a right to do? Where were my primary commitments? How would divorce affect the girls? I was afraid they would blame me for all the inevitable losses that accompany restructuring a family. I knew I would carry the brunt, because Roger wanted me to continue doing what I'd always done as his wife.

As I searched for guidance, the idea of a right decision gave way to choosing between love and fear. Though I was afraid of how the girls would adjust and how I would manage economically, my heart kept coming home to the love I'd felt with Andrew for more than two years. Yes, I loved my children and was committed to protecting them from pain, but if I didn't live in a way that honored my truth, if I stayed in a marriage that was in form only, what would they learn about being authentic themselves?

As I had feared, Roger was furious when I told him I wanted a divorce. How dare I disrupt what was working for him! As he absorbed the news, he alternated between rage and apologizing for what he'd said during the last argument. What love I still had for him faded as we both faced the truth of what we'd clung to and still struggled to let go.

I often speak with my clients about "leaving home" as part of their healing process, and that is what I did by asking Roger for a divorce. I broke with the family legacy — with what I had been raised to believe about being a woman, a wife, and a mother. In stepping outside the outlines of the roles I had played and assumed were my true and total self, I broke the rules that were meant to keep me safe, warm, and dry. Once I made my decision, there was no turning back.

Mother Load

If she could make it to the top
of the hill carrying her entire and
acknowledged load of sorrows
and mistakes . . . it seemed to
her she might be granted a kind
of spiritual second wind.

GAIL GODWIN

"He talks to me about his relationship with Celia," Erin declared in a defiant tone, turning her head to look at me from the passenger seat, as I drove her to one of her Nutrition Clinic appointments. "He treats me like an adult, but you act like I'm a child. I'll never have the friendship with you that I do with Dad!"

I stared ahead at the winding asphalt, my knuckles white from clutching the steering wheel. Roger and I had been divorced for over a year, and Andrew and I were adjusting to our newly created family.

"Regardless of what your dad does, I'm not going to discuss my relationship with Andy with you," I said firmly, sounding stronger and clearer than I felt.

I gripped the wheel harder.

Later that evening, as Erin and I watched a movie together, she snuggled against me on the couch. My sweetie pie was back, at least for a few precious moments, but I didn't know who the real Erin was.

Years later, Erin and I were at a coffee shop when she confided in me that she remembered how happy and confident she had been before she'd contracted rheumatic fever, and how hypersensitive and raw she felt afterwards.

"That's when I started stealing and trying not to eat." I realized then that despite linking Erin's difficult nature and mood swings with the divorce, it was in fact due to something that had been out of my control.

When Erin was only nine years old, in the first months of third grade, she had an undiagnosed episode of rheumatic fever. She had had a sore throat and recovered quickly, but shortly after her symptoms subsided, she seemed to trip more often and bump into furniture, which was very uncharacteristic of her. She had always been so coordinated. When I saw that her handwriting had deteriorated on the school papers she brought home, I made an appointment for a medical checkup. The doctor looked at me with alarm when she heard a heart murmur that hadn't been there before.

"I don't want to speculate about what this might be," she said.

I imagined her mind spinning through all the possible diseases and conditions, not wanting to say anything that might worry me more.

The doctor set up an appointment for Erin the following day with a specialist at Geisinger, which was a large medical center several hours away. "Try not to worry. It might not be serious at all," she told me.

Roger and I packed up all the girls and drove down for Erin's appointment the next day. After interviews and tests with several doctors, she was diagnosed with Sydenham's chorea, a disease caused by rheumatic fever that could become quite serious if left untreated. The doctor explained that Erin had had an undiagnosed strep infection that her body fought off. He said that the tissue around the brain and around the heart have a similar configuration to strep bacteria, and her immune system started attacking those tissues, which explained the heart murmur and neurological symptoms. Once she was treated with antibiotics, her clumsiness went away. The pediatric cardiologist prescribed echograms every month. Within six months her heart looked fine, and we were told she was healing well. No one suggested there might be any long-term neurological, emotional, or psychological effects. I had thought that chapter was closed.

However, we found out years later that there is a significant correlation between the development of Obsessive Compulsive Anxiety Disorder and Sydenham's chorea. Erin had always been a very sensitive child, but now that sensitivity seemed to be magnified 1,000 percent. The littlest thing would set her off, and she would sulk and snap at me and her sisters with little provocation. Andrew had always referred to her "Queen Anne's Lace temperament" to describe her sensitivity, and that temperament was even more pronounced after the rheumatic fever. Along with the genetic history of bipolar disorder in Roger's family and my family's obsession with thinness, all of these factors stacked the odds against her that she would not only be more susceptible to an eating disorder, but more helpless against it.

Realizing that something organic had prevented her from getting well despite the counseling, hospitalizations, and all our efforts to help her, was both a relief and a greater sadness. The injury to the "lining of the brain," as they called it at the time, seemed to have damaged her ability to contain herself, to keep negative thoughts, feelings, and behaviors in check. The shadow side of her ran rampant, while another part of her, like us, watched helplessly. And it was sad because it meant it couldn't have been any other way. She was the victim. I had seen her as a train that got up so much speed it couldn't stop, but instead, she had been hijacked by an invisible force.

We'll never know if it could have been different if we and the treatment experts had realized this at the beginning. What I do know is that "if only" is a bleak and barren path leading nowhere.

The link between her eating disorder and Sydenham's chorea was established long after the disease had taken over her body, and until that connection was made, I blamed myself for everything Erin was going through, including her mood swings. Though I once thought I was so strong and confident about my mothering, the girls' anger with me about the divorce and now Erin's prolonged moodiness and eating disorder had me questioning how good a mother I could have been. After all, if someone was mad at me, I must have done something to deserve it. I was the quintessential Good Girl, following the rules and never challenging authority. Approval from others was the mother's milk for my insecure ego. Even though Erin was a teenager suffering from an eating disorder, when her reactions were unpredictable and volatile, I took it personally.

I had a story in my mind about what it means to be a mother. I'd embodied the story from my own mother, who seemed to ask, like so many in her generation and before, "What's the next line I'm supposed to read?" rather than "What do I want?" I didn't know how to break from that powerful example without feeling inherently wrong or bad. I had broken the rules by divorcing my husband, and then Erin's eating disorder laid her down across the track in front of me. I couldn't back up, and I couldn't move forward. Maybe if I had just followed the rules, this wouldn't be happening.

Novelist Elizabeth Berg once wrote, "You are born into your family and your family is born into you. No returns. No exchanges." And so it was with me and mine. Do well in school, work hard, and don't upset anyone. Happiness will follow: a gold pot of delayed gratification at the end of the rainbow of ceaseless perfect doing. These were the unspoken family commandments that guaranteed the gates of a heavenly adulthood would open to me. Listening to your feelings and following your heart were for impractical dreamers. That's what my mother taught by example, and that's what I believed. When it came to Erin, I heard her voice in my head ask: *What did you do to deserve this?*

After all, I must have done something wrong to have so much pain. I wouldn't have tripped if I had been watching my feet. With my clients, I call the belief that I must have done something wrong to make a bad thing happen, or the flip side, that if I do everything right, all will be well, the "illusion of control." There is comfort in thinking that I have such absolute control — it keeps the fear of the arbitrary and unknowable at bay. We may know we're human, but we can pretend we're invincible if only we're careful enough, coloring between the tribe-drawn lines. I was falling through the cracks between stories, the story of who I thought I was and should be, and the new story that I was kicking and screaming my way into. I was losing my grip on my daughter, losing my grip on who I was as a mother. And my own mother, whose arms I longed for in these moments, was no longer there.

CHAPTER

Motherless

Nothing can make up for
the absence of someone we love,
and it would be wrong to try to
find a substitute; we must simply
hold out and see it through.

DIETRICH BONHOEFFER

It was a sunny Saturday morning in 1992. As I felt around the back of a closet shelf for spare vacuum cleaner bags, my hand brushed the rough brown paper covering a small square box. I knew what it was before I pulled it out from behind tennis balls and bicycle helmets. As I dusted it off, tears pooled in my eyes. I ached to go home and fall into my mother's arms, but instead, I was holding all that physically remained of her. My father had once asked me to keep her ashes and mix them with his after he died.

That morning I had awakened with a start, my heart pounding with panic and sadness, dreaming that I had only two days to live. How could I leave the girls and Andrew? Why did I have to die before having the chance to enjoy my life and find some peace? I stayed under the covers a few extra minutes, letting the reality that I was alive and well sink in.

Now, holding the box of her remains, I was tired of being strong, and I wanted Mom to hold me up — to stroke my brow and wipe my tears. She died before she ever got to rest, and I feared it would be the same for me. But was I grieving for something that never could have happened? I always acted so strong, so in control of myself and my life.

Odds are I would have protected her from worrying about me. Rather than finding comfort in her arms, I might well have pretended that I was fine. I remember coming into the kitchen more than once as a child to find her quietly weeping. She would dry her eyes with the edge of her apron and go back to cooking or washing dishes, saying nothing, self-contained. I knew that whatever pained her was private. In later years I wondered if she found the solace she sought by keeping the house in order and by inconveniencing no one.

She was the only child of immigrants who had risen from peasant poverty in rural Finland to become proud hardworking homeowners in a blue-collar neighborhood of Buffalo. My grandfather, a factory worker, was as frugal with words as with money. My grandmother was a daytime housekeeper and saved her wages to provide my mother with piano lessons, and eventually, college. Though she doted on her daughter, my grandmother would, at times, retreat into icy silence, leaving my mother to assume she was being punished for some unknown offence. A physical beating would have been easier for my mother to endure than to be cast into an emotional exile that could last a week. My mother became an expert at scanning the domestic horizon for any signs of disturbance in the atmosphere.

As a wife and mother, Mom's finely tuned radar continued to pick up the signs of any emotional turbulence long before the winds of anger in our household could pick up speed. Anticipating others' needs and soothing any upset was her forte.

When Mom was in her late forties, my father began pressuring her to retire and to put her mother in a nursing home in Florida, 1,400 miles away, in order to free them to travel more. Mom loved her job and didn't want to retire so soon, and my grandmother didn't want to leave her only child. These impossible choices left Mom barely able to breathe. Literally. She was diagnosed with asthma. The onset was sudden and the cause was unknown. I came to believe that the weight of those conflicting wants was squeezing the life breath out of her.

Like so many women and men of her generation, my mother learned to "make the best of it" and comfort herself with the knowledge that she was "exceeding expectations." Her happiness was the by-product of making the beds with newly ironed sheets and agreeing with my father on any subject that mattered to him. Peace came from the relief of forestalling upset. Absence of anxiety equaled happiness. But at what cost? I doubt she ever tallied the tolls she paid with her own soul to satisfy the needs of my father and grandmother. Even as she revolved around them, they were moons to her sun — two satellites relying on her to keep their orbits from colliding.

August 1981. I stood in shock with the telephone receiver at my ear as the disembodied voice from across the country told me my mother had been in a car accident and was dead. Unlike the day-to-day moments that flow together with fuzzy benign continuity, the realization that she was gone with no warning, that there was nothing I could do, froze that moment in time — unreal in its utter, unchangeable reality.

Roger and I had moved only a month before from Minnesota to north central Pennsylvania where he would be teaching at a small state college. This put us within a half-day's drive of both our parents, and I looked forward to having my mother enjoy her granddaughters more than once or twice a year. But before any of that could happen, she was gone.

I learned firsthand that grief is about the future that will never be, and that a broken heart isn't just a metaphor. The foundation I thought was as solid as granite simply crumbled. I stood at the edge of a precipice facing a future I could no longer bring into focus. I woke up to a world that went on as before — the same cars drove by, the same carillon tolled the hours, and the neighborhood children raced their Hot Wheels up and down the cracked sidewalks on our block. And nothing was the same. I could never go home again.

Night after night, I drifted in that netherworld between waking and sleep, as images of all the moments we would never experience played like the preview to a movie that would never be released — walks with the children, holiday celebrations, and heart-to-heart talks over the coffee we both enjoyed scalding hot. When Mom appeared in my dreams, I would try to stay suspended in that thin place just before waking reality, willing the dream to be real. With a throbbing pain that edged into terror, my heart ached from a longed-for future forever lost. There was no rewind, Wite-Out or do-over. No apologies or reparations. Only later would I realize the inherent solace of knowing it wasn't about me — about what I had or hadn't done or been.

Mom and I had just begun to plumb some emotional depths as I settled into adulthood. On the few occasions she and I had the opportunity to talk, I discovered a private, reflective world that she kept well-hidden when I was growing up. When she died, not only did I grieve the mother I had known and the grandmother she would have been to my girls, I also grieved the relationship that never had a chance to unfold. Like mother, like daughter.

Mom's death made me even more grateful that, during the first years Roger and I were together, I had made the leap into faith that eluded me in childhood. Though my beliefs didn't fit into a specific religious framework, I had come to trust in a pervasive and benevolent spiritual dimension that sustains and exists in and beyond the physical. Growing up I was taught that our rewards were on earth and not in heaven: belief in God was a comforting myth for those less rational and emotionally self-sufficient. Our commandments were simply: be nice, work hard, and always tell the truth. Death was just the end of life, neither feared nor anticipated. No heaven. No hell. No purpose beyond doing the best you could with the time you had. I wanted so badly to believe, but I couldn't get past the literalism of the family mind. "How do you explain suffering, injustice, and cruelty if a loving God is in charge?" Dad would ask. Given my limited background in theology as a child, I had no answer.

Seeking escape into imagined realms through books, I trekked to the library every few days to eventually check out every volume in the juvenile section about King Arthur and Camelot. In this world that was both magical and defined — the realm of Merlin, myth, and romance — I fed my hunger for myth and meaning. While on the outside I did what was expected, I kept my hunger for the supernatural and mystical to myself.

It wasn't until my early twenties that I was able to bridge the gap between empiricism and faith, thanks to my mother-in-law, Carol. She had gathered a following of friends and acquaintances who sought her out for numerology and Tarot readings, for which she never charged. I recall being impressed with the premonition she had about the invitation Roger received to apply to the criminal justice graduate program that neither he nor she had known about previously. As our daughters arrived, her predictions about their individual personalities and gifts proved to be uncannily accurate. Because I believed that she was truthful and sane with no ulterior motive, I will be forever grateful that she was there to help me cross over the river of skepticism without leaving my brain behind.

Though I would never say that I know why Mom died, I consoled myself with the idea that she had been released from what was for her the impossible choice to disappoint one of the important people in her life. Even in her death, she couldn't have created less of a mess — her exit was quick and probably painless. Dad and the dog escaped all injury.

In the weeks after her death, caring for my daughters helped me cope and move through the grief. I couldn't spend hours crying or staring at the wall. They needed me, and focusing on them kept me moving in the fast-flowing stream of life that comes with a young family. I had diapers to change, meals to prepare, and the comfort of daily routines. Carrying on, no matter what, was the legacy my mother left me. In our family relationships were based on adherence to routine and meeting expectations. We were cogs in a predictable wheel that kept turning, and we labeled that turning closeness and connection.

This initiation into heartbreaking loss was different from the torturously protracted grief I later confronted with Erin. After my mother's death, I didn't feel the gnawing ache of self-doubt.

Her death had nothing to do with what I had or hadn't done, and I wasn't plagued with the anxiety I felt with Erin day in and day out. My mourning was free of wanting to hide from the possibility that I had failed to be good enough or kind enough, or that I had even played a part in building the wall upon which I pounded.

7

CHAPTER

Four Winds

When you don't get a miracle –
as when you do – it is a startling
moment of deciding again where
you stand in the universe.

PATSY CLAIRMONT

Despite weekly therapy sessions and checkups at the clinic, and our best efforts to support Erin's recovery, she continued to lose weight the first year after she was diagnosed. Her body composition check at the Nutrition Clinic revealed that she was depleting muscle to the point that irreparable organ damage was likely. As Erin's biological parents and the primary decision-makers, Roger and I were called into a meeting with Erin and the medical team, at which Carolyn, the director of the clinic, explained her recommendations for an inpatient hospitalization. Our health insurance had pre-certified treatment for depression and anorexia at Four Winds Hospital in Saratoga Springs, New York, and Carolyn felt this would be a good choice for Erin because it wasn't overly regimented, had a program geared toward adolescents, and offered a variety of creative therapies such as art, dance, and psychodrama.

Erin, now 14, was quiet on the long drive to Saratoga Springs, despite my attempts to cheer her and make conversation. She had balked at the idea of being hospitalized, but like a dog that stops struggling against the veterinarian's prods and pokes, she seemed to have given up fighting the inevitable. It was a bright, hot spring day in 1991 when Roger, Erin, and I pulled up the circular drive in front of the administration building for Four Winds.

This looks more like a resort than a medical facility, I thought, as I scanned the red brick, peak-roofed, one-story buildings surrounded by lawns and blooming gardens.

We met with some of the staff and toured the campus. When I saw the art therapy room with assorted paints, pastels, large pads of newsprint, and clay, I watched Erin's face, naively hoping she would react as if we were leaving her at summer camp instead of this enemy fortress that wanted to take away the anorexia that had become her best friend and protector, her death trap sanctuary. But her eyes seemed distant, her expression blank.

After carrying Erin's duffel bag and schoolbooks to her semi-private room, I hugged her unresponsive body, and Roger and I returned to the car. I sank into the passenger seat, sighing with relief at leaving her in the care of professionals who, I told myself, could somehow find and recover the happy, confident little girl I missed. I should feel sad, I told myself, but having a few weeks of respite from watching and battling with her disorder felt more like the beginning of a vacation. My relationship with Erin had been so strained that I hoped the break would bring us closer together. Yet I was anxious, too, about what she would say about me in her therapy sessions. Would I be the target, the scapegoat, the one who unwittingly caused her anorexia? I worried about my weight, but tried not to show it. I exercised regularly, but hoped that it didn't seem obsessive. And, to top it off, I had divorced her father. Maybe it *was* my fault.

A month later, Jenna kept me company on the five-hour drive to bring her sister home. I put my hand over my heart, trying to stop the jackhammering in my chest as we waited outside the reception area for a staff person to find her. After several long minutes, Erin walked toward us down the brightly lit hallway, her face blank and closed. The joyful reunion I had fantasized about dropped with a thud into my clenched stomach. When I reached out to hug her, her arms hung limp.

Here we go again, I thought. *She's punishing me.*

As I scanned her frame for signs of some weight gain, I chattered about some happenings at home, trying to get some response from her, but she wasn't buying it.

Like a precious heirloom I had entrusted to the experts to restore, I naively hoped the happy girl I'd lost would be restored by daily therapy and physical distance from reminders of the painful past few years. Instead, I was carrying home a vase with crazy glue oozing from visible cracks.

After we met with the psychiatrist and I signed the discharge papers, the girls got into the back seat together. I hoped this meant Erin had missed her sisters and, despite her solemn expression, was looking forward to coming home. Years later, Jenna told me that Erin did mini leg lifts for most of the trip home.

"I didn't tell you then because I knew she'd be mad at me," Jenna confessed.

What I had passed off as sporadic episodes of sibling jealousy, I later saw as a breadcrumb trail I'd missed. I remember an evening early in 1982 when Roger and I had hosted a small gathering from the Episcopal Church. Erin was five years old, Jenna was three, and Ariel was a 16-month-old toddler — all safely tucked in bed by 7:30 p.m. before our guests arrived. As I served tea and coffee, we were startled by a scream from the room Erin and Jenna shared. Roger ran up to check on what was happening, and when he came downstairs he pulled me aside to tell me that Erin had gotten out of bed and pinched Jenna hard on her arm. I chalked up this small meanness to sibling rivalry. Up until then, the worst thing I knew that Erin had done was when, at age three, she'd cut off Jenna's blond curls with safety scissors. Later, I discovered there was a great deal more.

When I asked Ariel recently what she remembered about being afraid of Erin when she was young, she said, "I was about six and Jocie was only four, and we'd lock our bedroom door at night because we were so afraid Erin would come in and hurt us. She told me she had fantasies about smothering us while we were asleep, and that she wished we'd never been born. When we were a little older, she said that she wouldn't be sick if it weren't for us."

"Why didn't you tell me about this?" I asked.

"I thought you knew."

Several years after terrorizing her younger sisters, Erin told me that she'd had fantasies of getting a kitchen knife and stabbing her father while he slept. Perhaps she told her father she had similar thoughts about hurting me. For longer than I'd known, there was a dark side to the lovely, graceful girl who danced and drew and whose smile was bright and innocent as she held four-month-old Jocie in her lap for the annual Christmas photo.

CHAPTER

8

Pasta Patrol

Our suffering is our inability
to settle. Suffering is
believing there is a way out.

JOAN TOLLIFSON

As I cleaned up the remains of lunch one Saturday afternoon in
March of 1993, I noticed that the cream-colored bowl of leftover pasta I was planning on heating up for dinner was no
longer in the bottom right of the refrigerator. I started pushing
aside jars and wrapped leftovers to see if it had been shoved to
the back. But it wasn't there. Anywhere. My rational mind
went off-line, as my inherited anxiety about wasted food and
the suspicion that Erin, now 16, had absconded with the
missing macaroni, distorted its value and importance. I took a
few deep breaths and climbed the stairs to her bedroom.

She was sitting cross-legged on the floor drawing in her sketch pad when I walked through the doorway.

"I can't find the pasta that was in the refrigerator," I announced, as calmly as I could.

"I didn't take it, if that's what you mean."

Erin's jaw was set as she turned her head toward me. She seemed ready to stare me down.

"Why do you always blame me?"

Why indeed? I thought.

Unwilling to continue the interrogation without any evidence or an admission, I went back downstairs wondering why I even bothered to ask her. Even though I didn't believe her, I wasn't going to risk rupturing our tenuous relationship even more by searching her room. If I didn't find anything, I would look more pathetic than I already felt at being upset about a missing bowl of pasta. I told myself I was giving her the chance to come clean on her own, though she never admitted to gutting a new half-gallon of ice cream or peeling the cheese off the leftover pizza unless caught red-handed. I was reaching for the dim possibility that she would confess, which would show that she could at least be honest with me. Then she would be taking some responsibility, breaking free of the addiction enough to admit to her behavior, even if it felt out of her control. Or so I thought. Without truthfulness, I didn't know who I was dealing with and what was real.

Later that day, while delivering clean stacks of folded laundry to the girls' rooms, I noticed the unmistakable smell of vomit coming from the upstairs bathroom. She had left a clue, and I was back on her trail, ready to search for what I didn't want to find. I strode into her room and opened the closet door. There it was — the thick cream-colored ceramic bowl, now less than half full. I burst into tears. Though I wasn't surprised, I'd kept hoping that I was wrong, that I deserved her steely eyed assertions of innocence. It was only macaroni, but it was so much more. I could buy more pasta, but I had no currency to trade for her truth.

She was sitting on her bed when I turned around to face her.

"I wanted to use that for dinner, but the worst part is that you lied to me!"

She looked up from her drawing with a cold expression. Didn't she care that I was hurting and that her behavior brought us to this point over and over?

"Stop being my therapist!" she yelled.

What does lying to me have to do with my being a therapist? I wondered.

Nonetheless, I felt trapped. No matter what I said, she hid behind that accusation, as if being a therapist was incompatible with being a mother.

"And get out of my room!"

She slammed the bedroom door as soon as I was in the hallway, and I heard the lock click. My heart was pounding as I pulled my jacket out of the front hall closet and strode up the hill past the cemetery. A bright mid-afternoon sun cut through the cold March air, as the exercise started to calm my pounding heart. What could I do? My mind raced. No matter what I tried, I was playing emotional Russian roulette, and every chamber had a bullet with my name.

That night I was startled awake by a vivid dream I recorded in my journal:

I was shopping with the girls and Erin asked me about a bathing suit she tried on. She lifted her shirt and showed me a white suit with ruffle tiers from the chest to the waist — very uncharacteristically childish for her — and her chest was covered with short straight dark brown hair

up to her neck and over to her arms. She seemed unbothered, almost
proud of the hair. I felt so sad and thought of suggesting she shave to
at least appear more normal. I was also saddened by the flatness of
her chest.

She wore her disorder like the hair that covered her body in my dream, the ruffled suit like a part of her clinging to eternal childhood, believing that she could hide her distorted appearance. Though her face looked her 16 years, her body was stuck in time at 12. Once she started on the hormones prescribed by an endocrinologist to stimulate breast development, he warned us that her bones wouldn't grow past her arrested height of five feet. The possibility of growing was slim, at best, so we hoped she could at least have a body whose shape reflected her age. But there was no way her poor body could eke out a pair of breasts when the flesh was being slowly starved off her bones.

Our battle over the pasta was as bizarre and futile as I felt in that dream. I became a detective who cast my daughter in the role of the clever criminal that I could still outsmart. I wanted to connect with her, and I thought that I needed her to be truthful for that to happen. But she couldn't be. She was more invested in protecting her eating disorder than in a genuine relationship with me. The disease had a stranglehold on her mind, and I was setting myself up in opposition to that, putting her in the middle. My frustration and helplessness sent me into an action overdrive. I couldn't stop her, but I could keep her from "getting away with it," from thinking that she could deceive me.

I was feeding a power struggle, and as long as I did that, I sent the message that only one of us could win. I wanted us to defeat the disorder together, but that wasn't possible as long as she was in its grip. Like the kidnapping victim who, after an extended captivity, defends her captors, Erin would protect the disorder at the expense of our relationship. I reacted as if she were rejecting me.

I was so caught up in trying to control the situation — for her own good, of course — that I didn't see how I was making it even worse. If only I had been able to step back from my anxiety about wasted food, the money that was flushed down the toilet with every binge and purge, and, most importantly, the personal betrayal I felt when she broke agreement after agreement and lied to boot, I might have responded with more grace and less defensiveness.

But when I remember the central and even deified role food played in my life as a child, and how that was interwoven with my mother's restrictive eating patterns and my own weight-consciousness, I began to understand why it was so hard for me to know what was "my stuff," "her stuff," or an inextricable dance between the two.

In Food We Trust

Meaning isn't what
a situation gives us; it's
what we give to a situation.
MARIANNE WILLIAMSON

Whether or not eating disorders have a genetic component may be debated. However, those of us who work in the field of mental health often observe the powerful patterns that repeat from one generation to the next. The first time I took Erin to see the doctor at the Nutrition Clinic, Dr. Calderone, he suggested that Erin was predestined to develop an eating disorder at some point.

"If it hadn't been your divorce, something else would have triggered the eating disorder," he said. "I think she was genetically programmed for this. If you hadn't divorced, it might have been a break-up with a boyfriend later on. It was just a matter of time before something set it off. Don't blame yourself." I hadn't considered any influences beyond my example and my mother's perfectionist and driven temperament.

When I thought about my own history with food and my negative relationship to my body, I remembered being 11 years old, waiting with my mother in a pediatrician's examining room with the ubiquitous Norman Rockwell print of a kindly old physician holding a stethoscope up to a little girl's doll. When my own routine exam was over, the doctor had me step on the scale, sliding the weight to the right until it balanced at 112 pounds. My face flushed as the chart on the wall pronounced me a few pounds overweight for my five-foot height.

"I'd like to check my weight, too," my mother said, "just to see if our scale at home is accurate."

As she stepped on the scale, the doctor shuffled the weights to the left.

"One hundred ten," he said, looking at her questioningly. "Have you been feeling all right?"

"I haven't been very hungry because I've been a little constipated," she replied, the same line she gave my father if he happened to notice her scanty plate. At five-feet, seven-inches, she was underweight.

I had always been "a bit chunky," and now I felt even more shamed by my relative bulk — a prepubescent elephant with a gazelle for a mother. Though far from fat, I was nonetheless humiliated by my failure to be thin. Even worse, my own mother was thinner than me! There were very few overweight children in those pre-computer-age days.

I now believe my mother made herself thin and light as a covert rebellion against my domineering grandmother, who laced herself into a corset every morning before sliding on her size 16 housedress. In this passive, silent way Mom declared her independence. She couldn't speak up to my father, either, but she could control what she ate.

"Do you think the breast meat is a little dry?" Mom would ask, as the first slices of holiday turkey were passed. "I think the one we had last year was moister. Wasn't that from Bells? This one came from Tops. Maybe I kept it in the oven too long . . ."

How could she even remember last year's bird? Meanwhile, my grandmother gnawed on the neck.

"There's a little mashed potato left in this bowl," Mom might say, as she surveyed the half-empty serving dishes and cleaned plates. My father patted his belly and reached for the bowl with a smile. *Thou must never waste food.* A pagan deacon at the altar, my father finished the sacramental offerings.

Scraping edible food into the garbage was as unthinkable in our family as emptying your change purse into the trash. Though the monetary value of the leftovers might be pennies, they weighed like gold. Eating well was the antidote to my grandparents' legacy of poverty as peasant immigrants. Living through the Depression during their first decade in the United States only added to their ferocious obsession. Having the best quality meats and vegetables was their only indulgence. Reliable comfort in a fickle world, food seemed to fill more than their bellies. Little else could be trusted.

As a teenager I read every diet article and tried the latest exercise regimens advertised on television and in magazines. By the time I was 16, I had a calorie-counter chart tattooed in my brain. I packed mini-lunches — a dry half-sandwich with a side of carrots and celery sticks — but by dinnertime I was so ravenous that my self-control surrendered to the fat-glazed roasted carrots and potatoes that accompanied my mother's succulent pot roast and gravy. Dessert was a nightly event, with my mother taking half a serving, if she took any at all. Often she sectioned an orange on her plate while the rest of us dove into a warm pineapple upside-down cake dripping with whipped cream.

Jealous of her willpower and despising my weakness, night after night I determined to follow through on an extended fast out of which I would emerge like an ethereal waif. It never happened. With each new diet I vacillated between the smug satisfaction of self-denial and the angry self-loathing that took over when I stepped on the scale to find my weight had barely budged.

It wasn't until my freshman year of college, out from under my parents' watchful eyes and the temptation of those delicious dinners, that I conquered my demon. After a physical education class, I had stepped on the scale in the gymnasium locker room to discover I had gained seven freshman pounds in only six weeks. Those late evening dorm room snacks with my roommates hadn't gone unpunished. This time I was determined to succeed. I counted every calorie and began swimming every night in the Olympic-length pool. Two months later, I was thinner than I had ever been and logging a mile with every swim. For the first time in my life I enjoyed seeing myself unclothed in the dressing room mirror. I couldn't wait to go home like a conquering heroine.

On the drive home for Thanksgiving, I fantasized about my mother's eyes widening as she took in my newly svelte self, hoping beyond hope she would say, "You look great!" But she didn't. Perhaps she was worried, but she didn't say anything. What she said, if anything, I don't remember. And my father only commented on the diminished balance in my checking account because I had needed a new wardrobe in a smaller size. By Christmas I had dropped 15 pounds, and I was on a roll. My mental calorie-counter was on automatic, every bite tallied to keep me within my calorie allotment. And I kept losing weight. At times I got scared I might be losing too much, but I was more afraid of having my high school body catch up with me if I didn't stay ever-vigilant.

I'd also hoped that shedding physical weight would automatically shed my socially awkward self — the self that envied the girls who traveled in flocks, giggled in corners, and always had dates. I hadn't even gone to the prom. I had decided I would reinvent myself in college. And by the end of the spring semester — which ended prematurely when the administration decided to send everyone home with their standing grades as final to avoid a campus uprising after the Kent State shootings — I was thin and engaged to be married to the only boy I'd ever kissed.

During that pivotal freshman year, I had a quiet, sad-eyed, suitemate named Margo. She never went down to the cafeteria with the rest of us, though we invited her time and again. Thin arms and skinny calves were all we saw beyond the formless baggy dresses she always wore.

"I just saw Margo down at the vending machines stuffing an ice cream sandwich in her mouth. She tried to duck around the corner when she saw me," my roommate mentioned upon returning from the laundry room one Saturday afternoon.

We didn't know what to make of this, though clearly something was wrong, since we never saw Margo eat or drink anything but Tab. When Margo returned to our dorm room 15 minutes later, she went straight into the bathroom.

I don't know how I guessed that she was gorging on vending machine snacks when she disappeared for hours, only to throw it all up when she reappeared. No one talked about eating disorders back then. Diets, yes. Bingeing and purging, no. There were no Lifetime movies featuring starving teens and war-weary worried parents. A quiet wraith in our boisterous midst, Margo looked lost and sad, and I've wondered, at times, what happened to her. Even though I counted every calorie Monday through Friday, it was just a diet in my eyes. By the weekend I had earned a reprieve. I allowed myself a few slices of pizza, dessert after dinner, and, of course, a few beers on Saturday night. Perhaps that was my salvation. I couldn't do deprivation non-stop.

It took being out of my parents' house to realize that not all families make food the centerpiece of their lives. I was spending the weekend during my sophomore year with my future husband's family. Much of the food was processed, and I took a small portion of everything (except a slice of Wonder Bread), and was still hungry. I expected a homemade dessert, and instead Carol pulled out a package of Keebler marshmallow cookies. In my family we would have eaten at the dining room table with a lace tablecloth and using the good china and cloth napkins. My meager portions would have elicited concern.

"Aren't you hungry? Won't you have some more? You hardly ate anything."

But here, no one seemed to notice. We ate off unbreakable Corelle plates on the bare maple table with its worn finish, paper napkins bunched in a plastic holder next to the salt and pepper shakers. The mashed potatoes from a box and meatloaf disappeared into the cavernous bellies of adolescent boys. I was used to having every bite that anyone ate monitored by the Female in Charge. Here she happily surveyed her brood, oblivious to the lack of decorum and to my discomfort in this strange land where food was not God.

With each successive visit, I began bridging the cultural divide, appreciating the casual atmosphere, my future mother-in-law Carol's interest in knowing me, and her easy conversation. I even got used to instant coffee and appreciated the Oreos and ice cream that Carol and I often enjoyed together before bed while we talked at the kitchen table. Meanwhile, the male contingent was in the basement family room watching sports on television, their laughing and uninhibited shouts at a comforting distance.

This was not my parents' living room, with my mother nodding to sleep over a psychology book or *The New York Times Magazine* and my father peering over his newspaper at the *MacNeil/Lehrer Report*.

If not for the contrast of experiencing a family who didn't spend each day obsessing over meal times, I wouldn't have remembered the following brief conversation with my mother. Roger and I were visiting my parents for the weekend while we were both still in college. As Mom and I drove to the mall, she was fidgety as she gripped the steering wheel.

"What's wrong?" I asked.

"I didn't realize it was this late," she replied. "We need to get back. Your father will be waiting for his lunch."

Having been out of this context for a few years, I could see the craziness of her, a professional woman, allowing her activities to be dictated by my father's helplessness in the kitchen, as well as his inflexibility around mealtimes.

"He's a grown-up. He can get his own lunch!" I blurted.

"But I have to be there to feed him," she replied quietly, as she turned the car toward home.

I knew this would go nowhere, but I was brash in my no-longer-a-child wisdom.

"There's more to life than food!" I pleaded.

"But what else is there?" she replied, probably too quickly to hear the transparency of those words I would never forget.

Years later I battled with the fear that, because of this family legacy, Erin's eating disorder was my fault. I saw the generational obsession with food, my mother's "borderline anorexia," and my own fixation on exercise and staying thin, and I wondered if I had passed this onto Erin like a genetic disease. I wanted all my girls to feel better about their bodies than I ever had. I complimented them on how they looked and was determined not to weigh them down with the negative self-image I had absorbed from the worried look in my mother's eyes. I saw them as beautiful and told them so. But I didn't feel the same about myself.

I was trying not to be my mother, but I was born into her war zone with her body, and my daughters were bred in mine. I had thought my struggles with food and weight were over. Those early morning jogs gave me permission to eat healthy portions, enjoy the Tanqueray slushies at neighborhood parties, and I sincerely delighted in my girls' strong, healthy bodies.

Jenna once said she remembered me bustling around the kitchen at mealtimes, finally sitting down to smaller portions than everyone else. Was I more like my mother than I realized? I didn't remember myself this way. But I could readily recall my mother taking half of everything, from a piece of bread to half of a cookie for dessert. Like those television shows where you see an event through two different characters' eyes, I recall sitting down with everyone else and eating ample amounts. Jenna's version may be closer to the truth. Perhaps I was doing what I'd always done, much more aware of what I said than what I did. Those were the actions that out-shouted any words I spoke.

Deferring to my father and preparing meals were the organizing principles of my mother's life, and though I didn't see myself as revolving around Roger, I prepared every meal from scratch, baked our bread, and watched his moods the way I checked the weather forecast before deciding how to dress for work. All was well as long as I had meals to focus on, my children to tend to, and I was assured that my husband was well-fed.

It had worked for my grandparents and my parents, and for many years I believed it worked for me.

Belmont

There's a release in knowing
the truth, no matter how anguishing
it is. You come finally to the irreducible
thing, and there's nothing left to do
but pick it up and hold it. Then,
at least, you can enter the severe
mercy of acceptance.

SUE MONK KIDD

On a hot July day in 1994, I drove Erin down to Philadelphia for her third inpatient hospitalization. I remember sitting in the sunny admissions office of Belmont Hospital while the psychiatrist ticked off intake questions.

"And how many times a day do you binge and purge?" she asked, looking up at Erin.

"Maybe 12," Erin replied, matter-of-factly.

I gasped, but the psychiatrist seemed nonplussed as she jotted down the number and moved on to the next question. I'd thought two or three times at most. It was far worse than I'd imagined.

Driving home that hot afternoon, the seriousness of Erin's condition and her ability to hide how bad it had gotten slowly sank in. I remembered the tour of the eating disorder wing we had earlier that day, when she was introduced to some of the staff in the ward and shown her room. The nurse who led us through the bright sunny halls explained that every bite Erin ate would be monitored and every trip to the bathroom supervised. Binges and purges would be a thing of the past, I hoped, after what promised to be a stay of several weeks, and if determined necessary and approved by the insurance company, perhaps a month or more.

Whenever Erin was hospitalized, I knew she was safe, and others might succeed where I had failed in preventing her from doing further harm to herself. At least it was out of my hands. I could pretend to have a normal family life except for the phone calls every few days to check on how she was doing. What a relief after years of constant worry, frustration, and coming home to signs that she had stolen, binged, or vomited again. She wasn't my responsibility for a while and I could enjoy my other daughters with unclouded joy.

On that long drive home, I remembered a particularly painful day two summers before, when Erin's moods seemed like manipulations to keep me at a distance and protect her disorder. She learned that if she was angry enough, if she isolated herself in her room, I would give up and leave her alone. She had refused to eat dinner one night and retreated to her bedroom, where we didn't hear from her for the rest of the evening.

I fell into bed that night at 10, exhausted from the frenzied pace of our household, the frustration I felt at her belligerence, and a full day of clients at the Family Services Agency where I still worked.

Andrew and I were sound asleep by 10:30 when we awoke to her staggering into our bedroom, slurring her words as she said, "I took a bottle of sleeping pills two hours ago."

I wish I could say I leapt out of bed, gathered her in my arms, and reassured her that we would get her to the hospital right away. She had never threatened suicide, and I assumed she was not only depressed, but also wanting us to know how angry she was. I was angry, too, only aware at that point of how worn down I was by her erratic outbursts directed at me, and the fear and frustration I constantly felt about the daughter I had once adored. And now this.

"I'll take her to the ER," Andrew said. "If she can walk and talk, it's not too late. You can stay here."

Guilt and relief waged their familiar battle for my emotional center stage, and I sank back onto the pillow and lay there, my mind and heart racing for the next few hours until Andrew returned.

"They gave her ipecac and are keeping her overnight. She'll feel awful for awhile, but she'll be okay."

The next day, while she was recovering at the hospital, I had to take Zach, our long-haired gray tabby, to the veterinarian's office. He had been diagnosed with feline leukemia, and the vet had suggested it was time to put him to sleep. I cradled Zach in my arms one last time, tears streaming down my cheeks, before gently laying him on the stainless steel table. Within seconds after the vet administered the fatal shot, Zach closed his eyes and stopped breathing.

My chest was heaving with quiet sobs, and though I loved this cat, I knew I was releasing the fear and sadness I had been too tired, hurt, and angry to fully feel the night before. It was so simple with the cat — no expectations, no betrayal of dreams and fears about what would be next — an uncomplicated grief mixed with gratitude for the gift of his presence since he had appeared in our yard and adopted us a few years before. With Erin the love was always there, but overlaid with the tension of mutual hurt and warring agendas.

A week after leaving her at Belmont, I sat on the upper deck of our rental house on Hatteras Island, my legs propped up on the deck railing, enjoying the early morning sun as I wrote in my journal. We were relishing our annual pilgrimage to the trinity of sun, sand, and water, for the first time without Erin. Zane and the girls were still asleep, and Andrew was reading on the deck below. How could I put into words the mix of relief and guilt I felt at not having Erin with us? My life felt beautiful yet incomplete, like a set of heirloom china in which an irreplaceable plate has broken. I wanted to relax into the sun-baked pleasure of being by the sea, but thoughts of her hovered at the edges of my mind day and night.

I remembered the first blended family vacation, the summer before Andrew and I were to be married in September. We wanted to begin our stepfamily life on a high note, so we rented a house on the Outer Banks. Erin was 13, Zane 12, Jenna 11, Ariel nine, and Jocelyn seven. Erin had been anorexic and bulimic for more than a year, but we were still hopeful that with our love and support and continued treatment she would recover.

We left at midnight Friday in order to miss the rush hour traffic around Washington, D.C., and get to the vacation house by midday Saturday. The children were nestled with blankets and pillows in the back of the van and slept soundly until we stopped for breakfast.

When we finally arrived at the cottage, sleep deprived and achy from the 14-hour drive, we saw right away why we'd been able to get a house right on the beach for such a reasonable price. It looked like a shack that hadn't been renovated or redecorated in 30 years, with its worn yellowed linoleum and rust brown shag carpet. The only saving grace was having the beach a few steps from our door. The weather was lovely, so we stayed outside as much as possible, and at night we were lulled to sleep by the rhythmic roar of the waves — the only advantage to having no air conditioning.

One of our first afternoons there I was putting away the remains of lunch when Zane exclaimed, "What's with this?" I turned around as he dumped a newly opened bag of Oreos on the kitchen table. After popping one in his mouth, he had noticed something missing. He pulled out another, and then another. All the cookies had been licked clean of icing and sandwiched back together.

How could she think that we wouldn't find out? She hadn't even disposed of the evidence! Her invisible handicap became even more visible, and as secretive and manipulative as she could be around her bingeing or avoiding food altogether, we were amazed at how she left an obvious trail of crumbs. None of the smiling photos from that trip belie the frustration and helplessness from which there was no vacation.

Years later, as I sat on the upper deck of a lovely vacation house — pleasantly decorated, with air conditioning and up-to-date appliances — I wished she could be here to enjoy how far we'd come since that first trip several years before. But I didn't miss being at the grocery store and buying a bag of cookies, knowing that they might well disappear overnight — as would the leaf lettuce, cucumbers, and salsa, sans chips. I didn't miss seeing her pinched cheeks and bony hips, or the bits of chewed food under the rim of the toilet bowl. I missed the little girl I wanted to be with, the one who was long gone, replaced by a compulsive, volatile, and occasionally delightful young woman trapped in the skeletal frame of a child. I looked down at my legs as the journal rested on my thighs. Erin's legs were like mine — though stunted and bony, the only one of my daughters to be built like me. So this is how she would have looked.

On the last day of our beach week I woke up before dawn, pulled on shorts and a long-sleeved shirt, and headed for the sandy path through the dunes. Sadness at leaving this cherished place mixed with the anxious tension that was building in my chest about seeing Erin the next day. We planned to visit her at Belmont on our way home, and take advantage of the opportunity to have a family session with the psychiatrist. I had told her we would arrive late morning in order to spend some time with her before lunch, to be followed by our session at 1 p.m.

My mind was racing as I walked along the water's edge and watched the seabirds darting back and forth on the glistening sand. What if she can't stay at the hospital? What if she isn't better? What will they think of us arriving, tanned and sated by sun and saltwater, while Erin was in a locked unit where every bite and bathroom visit was watched? Will they see me as uncaring and insensitive because I wasn't at home, wringing my hands and calling every day? I wanted them to appreciate how hard it's been and would continue to be if she were discharged prematurely, and I was terrified we would end up back where we were before she was hospitalized if they did. Though I wanted to relax into the final afternoon of our vacation, worries about her buzzed at the edge of my mind, like an elusive mosquito in the dark.

Five hours later, as we approached the exit for the hospital, the knot in my stomach tightened. It was 11 a.m. when we pulled into the parking lot, the overcast sky mirroring my mood.

"Just wait here while we check on what's happening," I said to the four kids drooping among pillows and balled-up beach towels in the old gray Plymouth van. Andrew and I walked into the reception area to let the staff know we were there.

When the nurse came back from the unit where she had gone to fetch Erin, she said, "Erin has gone out for a walk with some of the other patients."

Like the quick flip of a switch, all my nervous energy became a current of righteous anger. I had told her when we would get there. Why wasn't she waiting for us? Part of me wanted to leave, another part to light into her when she finally showed up, probably in time for lunch. With Andrew trailing behind, I stormed out to the van where Zane and the girls were waiting.

"You can get out and stretch your legs, if you want. She went out for a walk, so we're not going to see her yet."

I tried to keep my voice level. After all, it wasn't their fault. Convinced that she was punishing me for another of my unnamed sins, I sat down in the front seat and pulled out my journal, hoping that venting onto paper would calm me down. After a few minutes I looked up only to see her walk right by me, flanked by six companions. Did she recognize the car and see me? If so, she didn't acknowledge it. In retrospect I could imagine how she might have struggled with seeing us heading home from a vacation without her. At the time, I was too swept up in the angry hurt of assumed rejection to have any empathy.

After getting some lunch at the hospital cafeteria, we all sat down in a circle of chairs with the psychiatrist in one of the group therapy rooms. Jenna leaned against Andrew's side with his arm around her waist, Jocelyn and Ariel, wide-eyed and looking unsure of what to expect, were on either side of me. Zane seemed subdued and curious, while Erin sat stiffly beside the doctor. After greeting us and introducing herself as Dr. Stone, the psychiatrist asked Erin if she was ready to speak. Erin nodded, opening up about how she dreaded her father's anger and never knew what kind of mood he would be in. She talked about the fear and shame she felt as a little girl when he punished her, and how confusing it was to have him cuddle her afterward and say he loved her. The psychiatrist noticed the other girls looking down, and asked if they shared some of the same feelings. They all nodded.

The psychiatrist must have read the guilt and sadness I was feeling in my face. "Did you know about this?" she asked.

"I knew he was disciplining them, but I didn't know that it was as bad as that," I said. "I wish I'd known and done something. I feel awful about it. Looking back I know that I was so afraid of upsetting her father because his temper scared me. It didn't even occur to me at the time that I wasn't protecting her. And I didn't know that he was as harsh as he was." I turned to Erin, and asked, "Do you remember when you were only two and you painted the walls and banister in Bemidji with Wite-Out?"

"No. Maybe I was too little. I hardly remember Bemidji at all."

"Well, I was typing your dad's dissertation and had just finished it the night before. Jenna wasn't born yet. It was one of those bright and cold Minnesota mornings. You were in your new bed, and sometimes you would get up before we did. You were always exploring and getting into things when I wasn't watching, like the night I found you in the cat litter."

Erin chuckled.

"When I came down the stairs that day I couldn't miss the small, white streaks all over the dark woodwork. You must have climbed up on a chair and gotten the Wite-Out off the table. It was still in your hand when I found you still painting on the top page of the dissertation. I freaked. All I could imagine was having to type the whole thing over again. Luckily you were only on the top page when I got to you. You dad must have heard me yell and he came running down the stairs. When he saw you holding the Wite-Out, he yelled, scooped you up, and ran back up the stairs. I thought he was just going to put you in your room for a time out. But I guess that wasn't all he did." I paused, waiting to see if she wanted to say something.

Erin was quiet, and the psychiatrist asked if there was anything I wanted to say to Erin, now.

"Just that I'm sorry. I wish I'd been stronger, I really didn't think he would hurt you." I looked at the other girls and said, "And I'm sorry I didn't check on what was happening to you, too. I didn't know, but I should have checked."

The psychiatrist nodded, "It's important for Erin and her sisters to know that you were still responsible, even though you didn't know exactly what was happening to them, and that you can apologize for not protecting them." I felt some of the guilt release, and as my eyes met Erin's, I saw understanding and gratitude in her face.

Turning to Erin again, Dr. Stone asked, "What else would you like your family to know?" Erin spoke of an incident at school when another student called her muscular thighs "fat," and how she couldn't get that out of her head. Once she started writing down everything she ate for the Life Skills class, it became easier and easier for her to eat less and less. Her mind had a will of its own, and hunger had little sway. She mentioned other wounding experiences, including her struggle with Roger's and my divorce. Even though she understood that the divorce was best for Roger and me, she hated the changes that went with it. She loved Andrew, but she wanted me more. "I know how busy you are and that you have to work, but I miss you! It's just not the same!" As the hour came to a close, Dr.

Stone encouraged each of the children to say what they were hoping for at this point.

"I just want her to be happy again," Ariel said.

And Jenna added, "I miss having a big sister."

Jocelyn said nothing, the tears rolling down her cheeks speaking volumes as she snuggled up against my side. Erin's face was soft and open, her shining eyes beaming relief and love. For a few brief minutes our shared disappointments and fears melted away, and we were simply a circle of love.

After the session we took turns hugging Erin goodbye before leaving for home. She would be staying at Belmont at least two more weeks. I squeezed her tightly, all the anxiety and anger that had been churning in my chest only a few hours before melted away by the sadness of how easily our individual hurts and fears could create chasms where we most needed to connect. The girls and Zane were quiet for much of the four-hour ride home. We had survived an emotional rebirth, the labor pains of revealed secrets bonding us even closer with the truth.

Therapy and Me

Good therapy helps. Good friends
help. Pretending that we are doing
better than we are doesn't. Shame
doesn't. Being heard does.

ANNE LAMOTT

Late on a winter afternoon in 1998 I was writing up my notes
from my first session with a woman who had spent several years
in therapy with Paula, the psychologist who had been Erin's first
therapist. The client had signed a Release of Information, so even
though I didn't feel the need for more background from Paula as
yet, I felt an urge to call. Paula picked up after the first ring.

I stated the reason for my call, and after a brief discussion
about the client, she asked, "How's Erin?"

"Not well. Terrible, in fact," I said with a sigh.

"I was afraid of that," Paula replied in her soothing, gravelly Southern drawl, her response both a surprise and relief. It told me that she must have suspected, long before I had given up hope, that Erin was unlikely to be healthy again.

"So how are *you* doing?" she continued.

I filled her in on the past few years, noting how I'd made difficult choices trying, often unsuccessfully, to keep Erin's problems and behaviors from controlling me.

"Listen," Paula said, "she's got to decide whether she'll beat this thing or not."

I didn't realize how heavy the pack of worry and self-doubt was until she lifted it off my back with those words. This professional, whom I respected and liked, wasn't telling me there was more for me to do, that I hadn't done enough, or that Erin's life was in my hands. I wanted to reach through the phone and hug her.

I remembered the first time we arrived in Paula's office, when Erin was 14. As we soon learned, Paula usually ran late, which left us plenty of time to fix a cup of hot cocoa or tea and help ourselves to the Pecan Crispies or chocolate-covered graham crackers that she kept on a side table in the waiting area. By the time she invited me into her consulting room, any impatience I felt dissolved in the warm bath of her presence — her intense gaze more comforting than threatening, her sharp intelligence focused on putting me together rather than taking me apart. I relaxed immediately.

During one of our sessions a month or two later, tears glazed her eyes as she shared that she had lost one of her daughters. Despite her professional success and her husband's successful corporate career, she knew what it was like to have a life that didn't go according to plan. Instead of casting Erin as a victim, she described her as an active and powerful player, making choices that mirrored her own hidden, even to herself, agenda. Despite, or perhaps because of Paula's X-ray vision, Erin trusted her, and I was comforted and confident that if anyone could help us as a family, she could. Unfortunately, less than a year into our work with her, she retired to write a book about family dynamics.

Not only was Paula a hard act to follow, but as therapists ourselves, Andrew and I knew several of the professionals who were recommended for Erin, and I was all too aware that anyone we chose would learn much more about me and my family than I might want to share with my colleagues. Erin was so bright and good at protecting her disorder; we needed to find someone who wouldn't be hoodwinked by her skillful defenses. She'd already had two hospitalizations at that point, and even with all the behavioral controls and therapy from inpatient staff who were experienced with hardcore anorexics and bulimics, her disorder had become more and more entrenched.

I thought we'd found a good match when we met Ann, a counselor in a town nearby. I'd heard of her and felt comfortable because she wasn't someone with whom we'd crossed professional paths. Though she had no letters behind her name, I was impressed by her bright mind and creative approach to therapy. She, in turn, was undaunted by the growing seriousness and complexity of Erin's condition.

Ann ran her therapy practice out of her home, her round oak kitchen table serving as the waiting area. We were invited to help ourselves to tea while she finished with another client. Although this in-home setting was unconventional and ran counter to the professional ethics of either social work or psychology, I brushed aside concerns about the fuzzy line between her personal and professional worlds.

Erin sat cross-legged in a large stuffed chair in Ann's office, her long bony fingers wrapped around a large mug of tea, while I settled into a wing-back chair in the corner between them. Andrew, more a supportive observer for our first session, sat across from me. Ann had her feet on an ottoman, a yellow legal pad on her lap, and her pen in constant motion as her questions peeled away layers of family patterns and beliefs.

Over the course of the first few sessions, sometimes with Erin and me, and several times with Roger or Andrew as well, it wasn't long before Ann's questions unmasked my self-critical streak, and I felt exposed and blamed for having been hard on myself. I wasn't good enough at not being too good. While Erin basked in the light of Ann's nurturing attention, I felt like a witness for the prosecution being cross-examined and misconstrued at every turn. Ann, the clever and relentless defense attorney, was carefully constructing the theory that Erin's illness was all, or at least mostly, about me. If I had been softer and easier on myself, Erin wouldn't have internalized so much perfectionism. My trying to be perfect was the flaw that Erin's self-doubt had fed on, so if I had felt better about myself, so would she. At least that's the story I heard, whatever Ann might have actually said.

When I brought up my fear, anger, and sadness in the face of Erin's bingeing and purging, lying, stealing, and emaciation, Ann told me to think about how Erin felt. In our world, according to Ann, the insecurity and shame that fueled Erin's eating disorder stemmed from her father's and my inadequate senses of self, in our individual shame and inherent personality flaws, which Erin had internalized and magnified. She was the victim of our imperfection, the pack mule of our emotional baggage. I shrank into the back of my chair.

So what am I supposed to do about that now? I wondered.
*You're telling me I've been too good at being good, and the damage
is done. I want to leave here feeling like I've done something right,
but instead, I feel like trying so hard to be right has been all wrong.*

"This isn't about blame," Ann said.

So why did I leave most sessions feeling frustrated, helpless,
and totally unappreciated? The very demons I was working so
hard to uncover and conquer in my own nature were blown out
of proportion in my daughter's psyche, and it seemed that none
of the good mothering I had done counted at all. I wanted Ann
to tell me that the nursing, rocking, and adoring care I gave
Erin as an infant had meant something, that dance classes,
encouraging her drawing, and tenderly caring for her when she
was sick or had scraped her knee mattered. But I felt like I was
throwing Styrofoam at stone. My deficits weighed in like lead,
while all the loving things I'd done barely tipped the needle.
Somehow it was my fault. I was making it all about me, and if
she was trying to absolve me, I didn't hear her. I felt both invisible and all too powerful.

After a particularly difficult session with both Erin and
Roger in which I felt targeted and misunderstood, I wrestled
with whether to continue in therapy with Ann. During one of
the earlier sessions Roger and I attended together with Erin, his
tearful apologies for the harsh and rage-filled spankings he
inflicted upon the girls brought tears to Ann's eyes. I, on the
other hand, felt like the whiny, complaining child she would
have preferred to banish. My grief and fear were distractions
from the attention Erin needed, and I had failed to be contrite
and apologetic enough about my failings.

Meanwhile Roger and Celia had begun seeing Ann for cou-
ples therapy. I questioned how Ann could be a safe place for
Erin to work through her hurt and anger with her father if Ann

was also counseling Roger separately, but I didn't know how to address that, or whether it was appropriate for me to do so. After yet another session in which I felt chastised and silenced, I decided to leave therapy with Ann.

Several weeks after leaving family therapy with Ann when I felt less raw, I wrote a letter to Ann explaining my decision. I hoped that she would hear and perhaps even acknowledge how I could have experienced the sessions as I had. I admitted my feelings of shame and tendency to be overly sensitive to criticism, hoping Ann could confess to her role in my experience.

However, when Ann responded, she said that she didn't see how I could have interpreted the sessions that way. According to her, it was all my misperception. I was wrong again. I wrestled with whether my rekindled anger with Ann was justified, and I tried to work through my feelings in my journal:

> I've been feeling guilty about the letter to Ann. Maybe it is all me. After standing up for myself so clearly, I'm now wondering if there are any flaws in my position. No wonder I have a hard time supporting myself. I'll never be perfect enough to deserve my own support. It's ridiculous! I have to live up to some incredible standard of flawlessness, totally knowing and sensitive, in order to be justified in my anger and in order to confront anyone. And I'm so critical now — ready to jump in and be annoyed about anything that doesn't go right. What a tiny, narrow window of opportunity I allow myself. The image comes of a small platform on top of a tall post — this is the ground I can take — so little space and so precarious.

I may have felt judged by Ann because I was so judging of myself. I believe she intended to be loving. She wanted to figure it out, find the missing puzzle piece that would complete the picture and explain why this beautiful, gifted girl with two good-enough parents was so sick and getting sicker. When she explored family history, I could almost hear the wheels turning in her bright, insightful mind. I felt like the unsuspecting pipeline for every past incident or trait that might have contributed to Erin's self-destructive behavior, the conduit who should have known how to shut down the valves to keep any of the genetic sludge from seeping into my daughter's psyche.

I needed my therapist to radiate the acceptance I had such trouble mustering up for myself. Though Ann always sent me off with a warm hug, the words I heard and the ones I wanted to hear bore more weight than her arms. I wanted her to say, "Yes, you were a wonderful mother. Yes, you did everything you could to give your children a better childhood than you had. And yes, it's not fair that this is happening. It doesn't mean you have been bad and are being punished. It's just happening. Let's see what we can do to bring more love, compassion, and understanding into this situation for everyone." But she didn't.

All healing begins with self-acceptance, the capacity to have awareness without judgment, and part of the therapist's role is to lead the client toward a more open heart with herself. Like a hungry mouse in a maze, I was frantically bumping into the walls of my own defenses and justifications, and I couldn't find my way out. I needed Ann to shine the flashlight on the exit sign of love and forgiveness that I couldn't see. And I needed to grieve — grieve about what was and might not be in order to soften to what is.

Years later, in reflecting on my experience with Ann, I remembered one of my early supervision sessions with a seasoned, gray-bearded social worker who came into the family services agency where I first worked. He listened to the case synopsis of one of my clients, an adult sexual abuse survivor, and said, "She's looking for confession and absolution." He taught me, in that simple, memorable phrase, that my client needed to tell her story in the light of day and see the acceptance in my eyes that she had not found in her own heart.

It was easy for me to see this young woman with compassion and no thought of judgment, to hear the choices she made as a child and adult as the natural consequences of what she knew and felt about herself at the time. Her "confession" didn't presuppose sin. It presupposed shame. That was the absolution I wanted from Ann. I was too full of grief and the fear that I had failed to give that to myself.

Erin remained in therapy with Ann for several more months. When I heard from Erin that she, Roger, and Celia had dinner with Ann and her partner after some of their sessions, any lingering doubts I'd had about my decision evaporated. Within the next year, after another inpatient hospitalization at Holliswood in Queens, Erin decided to continue her therapy at the local mental health clinic. She told me she'd become increasingly uncomfortable with Ann's close relationship with Roger and Celia and how that affected her trust in Ann's being able to help her with her "father issues." I had heard good things about a female therapist there who did very well with young women, and Erin readily formed a trusting relationship with Dana.

Several years before the Ann era I discovered a method for asking myself questions while journaling that seemed to connect to a wiser part of myself, a loving laser that cut through my conscious doubts and insecurities, finding an inner wisdom and answering questions that stumped my "normal" mind. I chose a green pen for those entries. Using that pen exclusively for the times I was reaching for help from another level often provided the guidance to me that I imagine I do when I'm at my best with my clients.

I decided to use that journaling technique to try to understand why I still bristled whenever Roger mentioned her name. So I asked, "What is it that still has a hold on me?" and my wise self answered:

Ann refuses to see you the way you wish to be seen. It may even be a power struggle over who will be the "good mother" and Erin's savior. Ann never had her own children, so all of her mothering energy gets channeled into her clients, who then must become her children. You are reacting on an energy level to Ann's attempt to mother Erin. "She has a mother!" you want to scream.

The more Ann acknowledges you as Erin's real mother, the more diminished her role is in terms of her need fulfillment. This is not a battle you need to fight. You are Erin's mother. Realize that Ann's need to control and take up a lot of space in this situation comes out of her need to be needed and her need to be seen as indispensable. Know that you are and always will be most important to Erin. There is no need to fight for recognition. Take the space that is yours with dignity and love, and do not move in or move out because of fear.

Good Grief

When you are sorrowful, look
again in your heart, and you shall
see that in truth you are weeping for
that which has been your delight.

KAHLIL GIBRAN

When I was a little girl I spent many Saturday afternoons with my father in his darkroom, watching as he dipped photo paper into chemical baths. Out of the shadowy forms emerged images of my mother standing at a railing with Niagara Falls in the background, family friends at a backyard picnic, my sister and brother playing hopscotch in the driveway, or last year's Christmas tree. A little red bulb glowed in the corner, providing just enough light for him to see what he was doing. I had been warned that opening the door could ruin an entire roll in a flash — a tenuously preserved past wiped out by too much light.

But now, in my adult life, the future seemed as fragile and uncertain as those developing photos. Who could have predicted that the lithely muscled girl in the black and turquoise bathing suit, who stood smiling on Jones Beach with the ocean as her backdrop, would, in the chemical bath of her disease, shrink into the skeletal version of who I expected she would be? It wasn't the past, but the future that was wiped out. As I wrote in my journal, I fleshed out those anticipated dreams, dipping the film of the once-expected future into the developer of my imagination.

I described the young woman she would have been if she had followed the "normal" course: a senior in college, probably a boyfriend, a career in the wings, or plans for graduate or art school. A blurry image of her grown to her genetically fulfilled height, an exceptionally attractive young woman with a sweet and sensitive disposition, wrestling with the usual yet exciting choices to be made at 22 — all this formed on the photo paper of my mind. Image after image of what would never be — a slideshow of hoped for and now impossible dreams.

I forced myself to feel and see her in that other possible life and make fully conscious the future that would never be. As long as I was focused on what she wasn't and wouldn't become, I pulled back even more from her, as if my denial of who she was and my resistance to accept her would somehow keep that other, desired daughter alive. I was afraid that by accepting her I would reinforce her current condition and give her a thumbs-up to staying that way.

For many years I had hoped that she could salvage enough normalcy to reclaim something of a life that seems to move forward and have some purpose other than struggle and survival, other than denying hunger, watching television, bingeing, purging, sleeping, and doing it all again. As I dipped picture after mental picture into the tray, I mourned the future I would never see, the daughter I would never celebrate. In my mind, I developed all the experiences that I had expected — for her to use and enjoy her talents, fall in love and marry, have children, come home for the holidays, share heart-to-heart talks about the joys and disappointments of life. And then I opened the door into the light that erased my fantasy film.

It was her never-to-be life, but it was also mine. I was grieving for her, and I was grieving for me. I don't even know how to separate the two — like the loss of a spouse is also the loss of the marriage and the loss of oneself as a mate. The evolution from mother to friend never happened. She was too needy and dependent, and I was too sad. How could I lay my head on her shoulder, when she could barely hold a bag of groceries without falling over? Instead of motherly pride when I saw her, I felt embarrassed to be seen with her, compounded by the guilt of feeling that way. I had to cry for the Erin who would never grow up. Was she in there somewhere, waiting to be released? Did she even acknowledge her existence? Perhaps that's why she started using Leah, her middle name, instead of Erin — it was too painful to acknowledge the child trapped inside. I, however, only ever referred to her as Erin.

Grieving was an ongoing process, weaving in and out of the daily pain, frustration, and helplessness of witnessing her relentless deterioration. I went into the local jewelry store to get a new battery for my watch one afternoon. Carrie, a former classmate and childhood friend of Erin's, was behind the counter. She was completing her student teaching and excitedly described her plans to find a job. As I listened to Carrie, everything she said reminded me of what Erin wasn't and might never do. I wished Carrie luck with moving and finding a teaching position in a larger city. I never pictured their paths so divergent when they played hide-and-go-seek as little girls.

Every major event in the other children's lives also became, for me, about Erin. What she would never be, do, experience. Even though I knew that I might never know why, I kept asking over and over, hoping that if I could make sense of this, even if I couldn't fix it, I could find some reprieve.

Erin's 19th birthday was approaching, and Walt Disney's *Cinderella* had just been released for purchase on VHS. I hoped that, like the fairy-tale spell that turned a pumpkin into a coach, a sweet memory of more innocent times could restore my daughter. Erin wasn't yet five when my mother died in 1981. Because of the geographic distance between us, they had had few times together.

During one of our summer trips home from Minnesota when Erin was two, my mother took her to see *Cinderella* in the movie theater. Erin wore her favorite frock, a blue-and-white calico shirtwaist with ruffled trim. The first time I tied the bow at the back of her waist, she said, "It looks like a butterfly, Mommy!" So from then on, we called it her "butterfly dress." When she and her grandmother got home from the movie, she burst into the kitchen, twirling and skipping to show me how she had spun and danced in the aisles.

This had been one of our precious memories of grandma and I hoped that giving her the video would reawaken that joyful innocence and ease the tension that was straining our relationship at the time. I wanted it to remind her not only of that special time, but of how she felt as a child when she asked to wear her "butterfly dress" most days until she outgrew it. She often said, "Remember the times I went to *Cinderella* with Grandma and danced?" As is often the case with children, the importance of that evening had registered in her memory as a repeated event.

I had made an angel food cake with strawberries, her favorite, and after we sang "Happy Birthday" and she blew out her candles, I handed her the wrapped videotape with a card describing my fond memory of that day 17 years before. She tore off the wrapping paper, glanced at the cover, and set it aside.

"Why don't you read the note, honey," I urged, trying to hide my disappointment.

She opened the card, read it to herself, and laid it on top of the movie without saying a word. No magic here. Familiar aching helplessness flowed into the space in my heart where tentative hope had briefly rented a spot. My body hadn't moved, but I wasn't there anymore. I didn't know what else I could do to connect with her.

Before she left to drive back up to Roger's house, where she had been staying for a few weeks, she took all of her artwork that we had framed off the living room walls. She didn't need to say why. I believed I was being punished. I had other children, a husband I adored, and a challenging career. I wondered if she was angry that I didn't put her on the top of the heap, making what she wanted from me matter more than anything or anyone else. At Roger's, she didn't have to vie for attention with anyone. I also believed that Roger had made progress in understanding the impact of his past behavior on Erin and wanted to be supportive of her. Staying with Roger for brief periods of time gave our household the respite we needed and provided Roger with the opportunity to offer what he could. So in removing her pictures, Erin took away what I had of hers that I valued. Even in the midst of my despair over her, those pictures reminded me of all that was still alive and beautiful in her — of her potential and creative life spirit. With the walls bare and with so much hurt over the past years, all that was left was the pain.

Locks and Lies

Don't try to put out a fire
by throwing on more fire! Don't
wash a wound with blood!

RUMI

It was 10:00 on a Saturday night in 1996 when the telephone rang. Anyone who knows us doesn't call that late, even on a weekend, so I assumed it was one of the kids' friends.

Instead, a male voice said, "Ma'am, this is the security officer at Walmart. We have your daughter here. Could you please come down to pick her up? She was caught shoplifting, and we can't release her without some supervision."

"We'll be right down," I replied, my voice flat as I tried to mask the frustration at having to clean up another of Erin's messes.

I was already in my robe and slippers watching a rented movie with Andrew. I ran upstairs and pulled on jeans and a sweatshirt.

She's 19 years old! When will she stop messing up her life? I wondered.

My heart pounded and my stomach was tight with guilt and anger as we drove down Main Street, dark and quiet this late in the evening. When Andrew and I walked into the bright fluorescent entrance to the store, a kind-faced older man I recognized as a regular cashier ushered us to the offices in the back.

When we entered the small gray office, the security officer was filling out some forms and Erin was standing to the side of a metal desk. She looked like a trapped animal, unsure of her fate, her eyes betraying fear of what our reaction would be. She seemed so small and scared that sadness for her began to overtake my anger and embarrassment. Even though she kept showing us how desperate she was, I still had trouble believing she couldn't control herself. Stealing from us was one thing, but being caught shoplifting was another.

"We've been watching her," the security guard said. "She's been warned before. She buys a few things, goes outside for a few minutes, and comes back in with her bag. She wanders around for awhile and then adds things to that bag and leaves without paying for them. It hasn't been anything valuable, just animal crackers, pretzels, stuff like that. We see how it is, but we can't let it go anymore. We reported her to the police."

In the end, she was barred from going into the store alone and she was put on probation. Although I wasn't protective of Walmart and knew that Erin's petty crimes weren't even a dust mote on their bottom line, I couldn't imagine her taking that kind of risk. Her fear of not having enough and needing to binge drove her like a junkie who robs his own grandmother to buy heroin. This was not a conscious choice involving conscience. And it didn't matter whether it was Walmart or her family.

Several years before, when Erin was 16, I was puzzled when I repeatedly found less money in my wallet than I'd thought was there. When I mentioned this to Andrew, he said he'd noticed the same thing. I had never worried about leaving my purse around the house any more than I thought about locking our front door. Then Jenna told me that her allowance money wasn't where she'd put it, and the change I'd left in a cup on the counter, once a mix of coins, was just pennies and nickels. I suspected Erin, but wondered if I were being paranoid. Andrew, who is rarely suspicious, said he had an idea. He marked a twenty dollar bill, put it in his wallet, and laid the wallet next to the computer. Several hours later when he checked, the bill was gone.

Meanwhile Erin had driven up to Roger's house for the afternoon. I called Roger, explained the situation, and he asked Erin to show him all her money. When she got out her wallet, the marked bill was there. A long, teary confession and apology followed, during which she admitted to stealing from everyone and agreed to pay substantial amounts back to us all from the savings account she had been feeding at our expense. I hoped that she had learned her lesson, but after that when we noticed our wallets were lighter and change was once again disappearing off the dressers, we began keeping our money out of sight.

A month after the wallet incident, one of Andrew's clients asked if we had experienced any theft in our neighborhood. "I had $200 in my glove compartment, and it's gone," she told us.

She had left her car unlocked in the driveway during her session at our home office. In those days before key remotes were commonplace, we usually left our cars unlocked, as well as our house, and never had a problem. Erin had been living at Roger's house for a few months, but she'd been at our house that day. We didn't have any proof, and Erin denied taking the money, so from that point on we suggested to our clients that they lock their cars.

I wanted to make decisions about Erin with Roger, but at first he interpreted that as an attempt to control him. He said that he felt criticized if we had differing opinions about how to handle her. When I saw his lips purse and tremble the way they had in the past before an angry outburst, I didn't shut down as I had throughout our marriage. I wondered if we weren't both shielding ourselves against being at fault while painting a bull's-eye on each other's back.

One Saturday afternoon Roger had stopped by the house to drop off a notebook Ariel had left at his house.

"Do you have a minute?" I asked.

"Sure. What's up?" he answered.

"I think Erin needs to go into treatment again. Her stealing is out of control," I explained.

His lips were pursed and trembling as he answered, "I'm doing everything I can!"

"I'm not blaming you," I said. "I can't control her when she's here, either."

He stepped back, dropping his shoulders, "I guess I thought you were saying that I'm not doing enough for her."

"Of course not," I replied. I knew that he had set up a separate area in his home for her, with a place to store her own food and have some privacy. Like me, he had hoped he could find some arrangement, some solution that would click.

"I know that I react to you the way I did to my father, expecting you to accuse me of doing something wrong. So I get critical myself and attack first," he revealed.

Moved by this admission, I said, "I get defensive with you, too, just the way I was with my dad. At the slightest sign of anger or criticism from him, I was ready and waiting, my armor in place and my verbal sword unsheathed."

Though it took years, I was grateful we were beginning to talk without blaming each other. And I learned that my resentment of him correlated with my inability to forgive myself. The less guilty I felt, the less I needed to make him wrong. We were learning to stop struggling and to stroke in the same direction as the current. It saved us a lot of anguish.

Erin was still living with Roger when I put pen to paper in my journal the day after her 19th birthday:

> We stopped really seeing each other, if we ever did, long ago. Instead, we see what's missing for us. She sees the mother I wasn't. I see the daughter she'll never be. What she needed me to be I don't know. I imagine her as a python, swallowing me whole — consuming, conquering, keeping me from ever being separate again, from being able to dance a different dance, alone, or with someone else.
>
> She said she was disappointed and surprised to still be alive on her birthday. When I hear that, it's like she's already died. We are both mourning her life. I'm feeling, in this moment, a level of compassion for her I haven't felt because I've been too consumed by my own pain — compassion for her being trapped in her body. I hear her silently screaming from the confines of her tiny frame, wanting to get out and so afraid, and I haven't been able to hear her. I needed her to be away from me for the sound to reach me.

Even though Erin was living at her father's, sticks of butter (to ease the exit of her stomach contents), cans of tuna, and boxes of dry cereal continued to disappear from our pantry. It wasn't so much the monetary value of all this, as it was the ongoing violation. Like Walmart, I had to draw a line. I couldn't do anything about what she was doing to her body, but I could at least keep her addictive behaviors from impinging on our household. Even though Erin wasn't addicted to drugs or alcohol, the drive to binge and have the money to do so was no different. It drove her to lie and steal to feed that overpowering need. It was as if she was in a trance — an altered state apart from her "true self." She couldn't stop herself, so we did what we could to stop her from both violating us and demeaning herself more. We changed the locks.

Andrew spent a Sunday afternoon installing a new lock on our front door, the only door for which Erin had a key. I was locking my own child out of the house. This thought banged at my brain like a puzzle piece you try to fit into a space where it doesn't belong. I was angry, and there was some satisfaction in being able to label my impulse to punish her by "setting consequences for her behavior." She paid for the new lock.

I felt sadly justified, knowing she couldn't get in without our permission (if we remembered to secure the doors), yet hated that we were locking one of our own children out of our house. It seemed nearly impossible to believe that there wasn't another way to reach her and to be "safe" ourselves. I wanted to connect with the part of her that was good and sweet and trustworthy, and be able to count on that. I knew she was ashamed of her behavior and felt increasingly ostracized from the rest of the family, but I didn't know how to include her without setting up ourselves, and her, over and over.

"We don't know what else to do," I said apologetically, when we told her about our decision.

"I was mad at you for going to the city without me," she admitted.

We had taken a weekend trip to visit Andrew's mother and had left Erin at home. We didn't want to exclude her, but when she had come to social events with us in others' homes, she hovered around tables of food as if in a trance, loading her plate with shrimp and other delicacies, oblivious to appropriate portions and ultimately purging it all. Purses left in bedrooms and wallets in coat pockets were likely targets, as well, and I wasn't willing to be her personal gendarme.

For awhile I was relieved to come downstairs in the morning and open the refrigerator or poke through cupboards for dinner ingredients without automatically scanning to see what was missing. Normal felt so nice. Yet she was always on my mind, even while I slept. I would awaken throughout the night with images of her pale and bony face. I wanted her to live with us, but I couldn't live with who I became when she did.

No matter what boundaries I set or aspects of our physical life we managed to secure from Erin's behaviors, I was constantly questioning myself. An unsettled, sick feeling in my stomach like the nausea I had during the early months of pregnancy accompanied any thought of her. I wasn't at peace, no matter what I did or said about what I did. As I explored this in my journal, I began to see that the only question worth asking was "Who do I want to be with her?" I couldn't control how she saw me, but I could control how I saw myself. I had given up my power to see myself except through how I imagined she saw me — as selfish, uncaring, and angry. In her eyes, through mine, I had no footing. I was never sure of myself.

I was caught in a web of accusations and defensiveness woven by my fear of having failed her and my grief over how she had failed me. Erin's lying and deception felt like manipulation and betrayal, and I didn't know how much was being driven by addiction and mental illness, and how much she could control if she wanted to. In my mind she was fighting to keep her eating disorder, and I was fighting to free her from it. The more out of control she was, the more out of control I felt. I assumed that other parents, at least the good ones, had control and knew what to do.

I assumed that my life as a mother would get easier as the girls became more independent, and that we would transition into mutually appreciative and supportive relationships. But instead of getting easier, my life was increasingly eclipsed by Erin's needs and behaviors, and even more so by my uncertainty about where and how to draw the line between what was my responsibility to her, for her, and to myself.

As Einstein once said, a problem is never solved at the level at which it is created. Because of that I couldn't problem solve my way to an action plan that worked. Erin's reality shifted with the winds of her illness, blowing away my hope for a solution.

Snapshot

Thus mired and bound I groaned aloud: nothing is loathsomer than the self-loathing of a self one loathes.

JOHN BARTH

Erin and I are sitting at a window table in a bustling restaurant two doors down from the office where Andrew and I work. I thought she would enjoy having a dinner out with me after our first meeting with a new psychiatrist. Her head is bowed over the menu as she flips through the pages.

Please order something other than dry salad, I mentally beam in her direction.

I look down at the open menu in front of me, pretending to ignore her. But I can't.

"So, honey, what do you think you'll have?" I ask brightly.

"I'm not sure yet," she answers, which I'm sure is code for, "I don't want to tell you."

After all, she must have memorized the menu by now.

Relax and leave her alone! I scold myself.

But I can't pretend that it doesn't matter to me what she orders. How many times have I sat across from her in a restaurant as she picked at a bowl of lettuce dressed with salsa? I have a right to be concerned! After all, if she were an alcoholic would I sit silently by while she ordered a beer, which, by the way, I paid for? But my irrefutable logic can't soothe me. If I say something, she'll get mad and be even less likely to order real food.

I notice another mother and daughter at a table against the wall. The pony-tailed daughter is dipping her French fries into ketchup and popping them one after another into her mouth in between sips of Pepsi as she listens to her mother, who is leaning forward over a half-eaten cheese steak sandwich.

Why can't we be like that?

"Are you ready to order?" the server says, snapping me out of my sad little reverie.

"We need a few more minutes," I answer, and she walks over to another table.

And then I realize I haven't picked anything, either. Out of habit I zero in on the entrée salads: spinach with hot bacon dressing, grilled chicken Caesar, taco salad with beef or chicken. I've had them all, dressing on the side, of course. Maybe I should order a sandwich to show Erin that it's okay — that I can be free with food. But I really do like salads. Or have I just convinced myself that that's what I should have? I want Erin to want something other than a salad, but if I order a salad, isn't that giving her more permission to do the same?

Aaaaargh!

I'm a pathetic Charlie Brown with Lucy trapped in my skull.

15

Pathfinders

Conscious freedom is the freedom to
meet suffering consciously, and then
consciously to let it go. The bondage is
in being unaware of the choice.

GANGAJI

"There's a new facility called Pathfinders in California that looks like a good possibility for Erin," suggested Carolyn, the director at the Nutrition Clinic, when I spoke with her in March of 1995 about what the next treatment steps might be for Erin. "They specialize in eating disorder treatment and offer all sorts of innovative and creative approaches to therapy, so it looks like a good fit."

"That sounds great!" I said, buoyed by the hope that these experts might finally break the stranglehold anorexia and bulimia had on Erin's brain and body.

Erin was 19 and blessedly still covered by her father's excellent health insurance. The clinic pre-certified the insurance coverage and arranged for her admission to Pathfinders. Roger and I split the cost of the airplane travel, and Erin flew to California for another inpatient hospitalization.

Every time I called to speak with Erin the first few days after she arrived, she was involved in an activity and unavailable to come to the telephone.

When I finally reached her therapist, Robin, she said, "Erin did a lot of work today. It would be best if she had control over making her next contact with you."

My face was instantly hot, as if she had reached through the phone and slapped me.

So she's working on her issues with me, no doubt, I thought.

I imagined my competent good therapist/good mother identity stripped from me, as I stood emotionally naked in front of the staff at Pathfinders. I imagined Erin criticizing me to the staff, distorting and defiling all my good efforts and intentions, and revealing only my fears and obsessions. I felt defenseless and exposed. In my fantasy I saw Erin as the gloating victor, hanging her discarded pain on my carcass, as if unmasking me freed her from the worst in herself, and her salvation would come by pushing me away as far as possible. I knew much of this was my projection, but when I couldn't speak to her, it was hard to let it go.

I had learned that Pathfinders offered on-site training for therapists, and I had considered flying out both to visit Erin while she was there and to participate in their week-long professional workshop. The day after I spoke with Robin, she left a message saying I could not come to the seminar in May while Erin was there. The staff had decided that my dual role as a professional and a mother would be counterproductive. Though I understood, I felt angry and hurt, as if I were being reprimanded or told I wasn't good enough. Meanwhile Erin hadn't called or written. Even though Robin said that Erin's not contacting me was a move toward independence, I felt rejected. The next morning, Andrew said he'd had an intuitive image of Erin wanting, more than anything, to be held by me like a baby, totally contained in my arms. I wondered if that might be why she needed so desperately to prove to herself that she could live without me.

Erin had been at Pathfinders for over a month when I awakened from a nightmare at 4 a.m. and couldn't get back to sleep. The terror in my dream echoed the anxiety I felt about seeing her in just six hours, when her flight home was due to land. I would be picking her up from the local airport and taking her straight to the hospital near the Nutrition Clinic. Not only had the program failed to help her, but Robin had called the day before to tell me that Erin's weight was down to 72 pounds, 27 pounds less than her once healthy, pre-disorder size. I was afraid to see her, unable to imagine how she could be even thinner. I thought the 80 pounds she weighed when she left was awful. Angry with Pathfinders and afraid of what it meant that one of the reputedly best facilities couldn't help her, I got out of bed, went downstairs, and filled the teakettle. While I waited for it to whistle, I gazed at Oreo, our long-haired feline ball of black and white fur, alternately licking and being licked by Tweeter, our wiry little orange huntress. Watching the cats and sipping my hot, milky sweet tea slowed the current in my chest, providing a wave of peace in a whirlpool of worry.

From a distance, I recognized Erin's walk as she approached along the arriving passengers' corridor in the airport. More bone than flesh, her smile a skeleton's grin, I swallowed a cry of shock and horror and held on tight inside as I hugged her. She looked worse than I had even imagined. I felt waves of fury with the psychiatrist and therapist who had allowed her to deteriorate to this point. How could they let this happen? As we walked to the baggage claim, I held her close to my side, ignoring the stares of the other travelers and greeters. I didn't dwell on what they might be thinking. She was alive. I loved her, and all I wanted was for her to get well. Her deterioration heightened both my feelings of helplessness as well as my desire for her to live, and to want to.

"How was the trip?" I asked, trying to keep the tension out of my voice.

"I went into some bookstores at the airport and had some chicken and salad for lunch on the plane," she replied, playing along with the attempt to make this seem like a normal mother-daughter reunion.

I collected her bags and carried them for her. I didn't want her to use up what little strength she might have left. As we drove to the clinic, I related her sisters' activities over the past month, my chatter an attempt to cover up the panic that was building as I snuck glances at, yet didn't want to see, her emaciated little body.

When we walked into the clinic waiting room, a heavyset woman was sitting with her young adolescent daughter. She looked up at Erin and me, raising her hands and eyebrows with helpless camaraderie, and said, "Kids!" She captured all and nothing in that quick exchange, as if the starving young woman by my side were having a typical teenage crisis. I nodded an acknowledgment, grateful for the attempt to understand.

Carolyn hurried out from her office to greet us, and when Erin went into the restroom, I fell into Carolyn's arms, sobbing and oblivious to anyone else there. Carolyn had been with us from the beginning, having founded the Nutrition Clinic only two years before we first brought Erin to her. The clinic offers the most comprehensive physical assessment and monitoring of individuals with eating disorders anywhere within hundreds of miles. Carolyn diligently coordinates treatment with other professionals, and researches and recommends inpatient treatment facilities when she believes a patient's physical well-being is at risk. She had monitored Erin's physical as well as emotional status from the outset, more than six years earlier, and had been a reassuring, non-blaming presence, as well as a reality check for my fears. I trusted her completely.

Carolyn weighed Erin and did a body composition test to check her fat/lean ratio and metabolism.

"I'm calling the hospital. Her levels are so low that we need to get her on IV fluids right away." I felt relieved to have Erin in responsible hands, yet stunned that she could have been allowed to regress so much.

"You can take her right over," Carolyn said when she got off the phone, and within minutes we arrived at the intensive care unit.

As Erin changed out of her clothes into the hospital gown, I felt a wave of nausea at the sight of her bare limbs and the meager outline of her torso through the thin cloth. What happened to all those promises of help and healing? How many more hospitals can there be? How many more failed treatments will she survive? That night her skeletal face haunted my dreams and penetrated the positive images I tried to focus on instead. There was no escape, even in sleep.

The next day I brought Jenna and Ariel to visit Erin. We strode down the antiseptic-smelling hospital halls, following the signs for the intensive care unit. Jenna, tall and blond, wearing athletic shorts and a basketball tournament T-shirt, striding beside Ariel, who sported newly red hair, jeans, and high-heeled sandals. The girls and I didn't speak, as if each of us were bracing for an unpredictable challenge. I wished we were headed for the mall or a long walk down the bike trail instead. Jenna had to leave for a basketball tournament that afternoon, Zane's high school graduation was the next day, and I was thinking about all the party preparations before family and friends arrived.

As we entered the large double doors to the ICU, I spotted Erin's bed straight ahead in a little curtained cubicle with inexplicable blinking and beeping machinery all around. She smiled at her sisters and averted her eyes from me. Now what? I had no idea what had prompted her change in attitude toward me since the day before. I wondered what it was like for her to be lying in this bed watching her tall, healthy sisters approach. Did she feel jealous, sad, or somehow triumphant? She pulled Jenna aside, whispering to her and twisting her body away from me. A pang of hurt shot through my chest at being so obviously shut out. As I took a deep breath, collecting myself, I felt a tap on my arm and turned around to see the hospital social worker.

"Can you step over here with me to look at some papers?" she asked.

I was relieved to be away from the tête-à-tête that excluded me and to have something else on which to focus. When we finished reviewing the forms, I went back to the foot of Erin's bed.

Ari whispered, "Jenna was hungry, and Erin gave her a can of Ensure."

I felt a flash of anger.

How can Erin sabotage her recovery like this! After all that is being done to help her, to save her!

Keeping my voice calm and looking directly at Erin, I said, "Did you ask Jenna to drink your Ensure?"

"Fuck you!" she spat at me.

The social worker was still standing there, looking awkwardly from one of us to the other. My face burned with embarrassment, anger, and hurt, and the steel doors around my heart clanged shut. I said nothing. The girls visited for another 30 minutes, which felt like hours. Erin's lunch arrived, providing an opening for us to leave. I leaned over, stiffly hugging her goodbye and rode an adrenaline current of helpless anger back down the bright, beige hallway, an image of Erin's defiant, rejecting face taunting me all the way home.

Only 24 hours before all I'd wanted was to envelop her with love and infuse her with the will to live that seemed to erode with every rejected pound. And now I couldn't stand to look at her. She had lashed out at me with such sudden venomous hatred, a counterpoint to my controlled emotional containment. It was so much easier to be sad and scared for her. I was still the Good Mother then, soft and full of loving concern. But in my righteous fury, all I wanted was to forget her, to have her out of my life. Even though those anger-driven thoughts didn't last, I felt guilty that they happened at all.

16

CHAPTER

The Picture of a
Thousand Words

Pain can burn you up and destroy you,
or burn you up and redeem you. It can
deliver you to entrenched despair, or
deliver you to your higher self.

MARIANNE WILLIAMSON

Erin had been living with Roger when, only two months after
her return from Pathfinders, another inpatient hospitalization
was arranged, this time in Pittsburgh. Because she was over 18
and not a full-time student, her father's health insurance, which
had paid for all the prior hospitalizations, no longer covered
her. I was grateful that a hospital social worker had arranged for
Erin's treatment to be covered by Medicaid.

The county also had arranged for a caseworker to drive her
the five hours to Pittsburgh, so I asked her to stop by before she
left. When I opened the door, she walked in without responding

to my forced cheery, "Hi, honey!" greeting. She didn't look at me, and her determined movements screamed anger.

About what? That I'm not driving her myself?

Nothing was normal, or as it should have been between a mother and daughter anymore. When had I last looked forward to seeing her and being with her? I smiled at and hugged her sisters eagerly and often. She had to see that — feel the difference between my loving lightness and the ease I poured into them, and the restrained, measured drops of attention I had for her.

She folded herself into a chair, bone too close to bone, all the flesh that should cushion and give shape to her limbs sacrificed ounce by ounce to the insatiable anorexia, like a tapeworm in her brain. Her ribs were diagonal ridges visible through the thin fabric of her second-hand child-size summer top. Adult clothing, no matter how small, didn't fit right.

I forged ahead.

"So . . . are you packed and ready to go?" I asked, as if she were leaving on a long-anticipated vacation.

Though she looked as if she could crumble like a dry leaf at the slightest touch, her voice was hard and challenging.

"I gave all my pictures that were in the coffee shop away," she said, ignoring my question. We had helped her frame a number of her pen and ink and colored pencil drawings, which had been displayed for several months at the coffee shop. She had hoped to sell some of them.

Her words, like an incendiary prepared speech, dropped into the space between us — a space that had become a minefield. For the past month there hadn't been any innocent, easy words for us. Even an inflection or tone might set her off, and we had to watch everything we said around her.

"You gave away the one I love? My favorite, of the tree? You know how much I love that picture!" My cheeks were burning. Though she didn't say it, I knew I was being punished.

She was angry with me, and I with her. We had let each other down, she by not being the child I could celebrate, and I by not being the ever-available mother. Eight years of anorexia and bulimia had worn down both of us, and I was weary and wary of being alternately reached for and then pushed away. Lying, stealing, and the painful sight of her body becoming more bone than flesh had taken its toll on my heart. Was this the fourth or fifth hospitalization? I had lost more hope when she returned, time after time, only to resume her starving and bingeing, denying and grasping for food just like she shut me out and yet longed to be enfolded by my maternal embrace. But throughout all of that, at least she and I had still celebrated her artwork.

Ever since she was a small child she had escaped into drawing, spending hours absorbed in intricate designs and fantasy images, and I found solace in the beauty she created. Colored pens in hand, she would be absorbed for hours creating images that seemed to come from another realm. This was the one part of her that was still intact, the one healthy thread that held strong even as the fabric of her life as I had imagined it would be — strong, bold, and bright — was torn to shreds.

The drawing I loved most is a colored pen and ink drawing of a mystical tree, in which fluid leafless amber limbs are wound with green Christmas lights reaching toward the risen sun in the upper right corner, with an equally large full moon perched lower behind the curling branches to the left. A shining planet rests at the tip of one bough in between, and roots wind into the ground, fully visible, flowering beneath the earth.

Like all of her drawings, I saw more each time I looked — an elaborate fairyland of miniature cats and snakes, stars and whimsical snails. Life celebrating itself — playful creation bursting into beauty beyond what could meet the physical eye. This was the child I remembered and missed, and I held onto the hope that if she could draw this way, she might still be in there. Though there was no space in her body, her spirit exploded onto the drawing pad, and I wanted that precious piece of her that I could still celebrate and touch with joy.

As she got older, her drawings became more and more detailed and symbolic. She tapped into a private world of snakes and stars and intricate designs, weaving representational forms with fantasy and archetype. Those images seemed to capture the paradox of her anorexia and bulimia — the powerful high and ultimate control as she transcended the needs of her physical body, and the dark helpless descent as her body inevitably rebelled and she crawled back, pulled down by her body's rebellion and shame, to the altar of her addiction. There she made her ritual sacrifices, placating the demon-disorder and reinforcing her fate. The snakes in her drawings appear harmless, wound around trees or superimposed on a serene female face, while the stars intermingle with tears. She could not imagine life without the disorder, but with it she would surely die.

But here, in her three-dimensional world, her voice was flat as it floated above my hurt and anger: "You could have paid $250 for it if you liked it that much."

I was screaming in my head, *I'm your mother! I've paid a far bigger price for you over and over. Years of therapy. Thousands of dollars of purged food. Pain beyond any price. And you gave my picture away!*

Out loud, in a tone as deliberate and disembodied as hers, I said, "I'm really hurt and angry. That picture meant a lot to me."

My exterior calm belied the adrenaline racing through my body. I have read stories about mothers who lift cars off their children, and in this moment I could have heaved a truck. But there was no physical way I could save her or fight her. I wanted hand-to-hand combat to wrestle away the insidious disease that had a death grip on her mind and free will, not this mock battle jabbing into thin air.

She repeated, "You could have bought it. . . ."

I said nothing and instead felt myself give up. We were sparring with each other over our mutual disappointment and anger. Did she do this deliberately to hurt me? If she wanted me to beam love at the part of her that danced with the demon, I couldn't do it. So, in return, she held back the part of her I longed for. Her anger gave me the message that she had control, but that may have been an illusion. Perhaps punishing me kept her own feelings of helplessness at bay, another sacrificial pound of love to feed her ravenous addiction.

As she unfolded herself slowly and walked to the door, each careful step seemed to state, "I'm in control here." Her goodbye sounded as hollow and restrained as our exchange. Would she even live until Thursday morning, when she was scheduled to leave? How could I feel so detached as I wondered about her possible death? She had to know how offended I was, but her steely stance and modulated voice didn't acknowledge my feelings, as if she were refusing to land in my turf by not engaging or responding to the intensity of my hurt. I had a brief fantasy that once she was away, I would find the woman she gave "my" tree picture to and ask for it. I was her mother, after all.

By the next day, when my heart was no longer pounding and anger had given way to the deep and constant sadness that accompanied all thoughts of her, I was relieved that she was leaving for the hospital — relieved that once again she would be safe and far away, where I wouldn't have to suppress the horror of seeing her.

I was afraid to hope, or to feel much at all, or maybe I was numb. Had my once unshakable devotion shriveled up with her body? Or was I simply waiting to see if I could invest more of my love, hope, and dreams into my precious, promising child who was imprisoned in a cage of ribs? If she died, would I cry? Or would I wander through the next days and weeks, absorbing my identity as a mother whose child has died, waiting for an emotional release like a dried up stream longs for a thunderstorm, longing to feel something, to have a torrent of grief rush through the banks of my body, cleaning me out, making it all palpably real?

In August, Andrew and I returned with Erin's sisters and Zane to Hatteras Island. After arriving at our rental house and unloading the car, I took my annual virgin walk along the shore. The beach was quiet, the sea a shimmering teal reflecting the deepening blue of the late afternoon sun. I longed for the Erin I expected when I had taken that picture of her at Jones Beach a decade before — the daughter I'd had no doubts I'd enjoy strolling with along the beach for years to come. That mental photograph, forever undeveloped, was replaced by my last image of her — an emaciated embodiment of alternating sadness and rage. She nearly died when she arrived at the hospital, we were told. Her potassium level was so low they said it was a miracle she survived, especially with such a devastated body. When I was finally able to speak with her the night before we left, she sounded so sad about not being with us that I felt sad too, for her and for us. She had been hospitalized for more than five weeks.

At the end of the month, we picked Erin up from Pittsburgh after helping Jenna move into her freshman dormitory room at a state university near the city. That night, in a darkened motel room north of Pittsburgh, Erin, Ariel, Jocelyn, Andrew, and I watched in stunned silence as the news reports of Princess Diana's death indelibly burned the calendar date in my mind. Erin, nearly 21, was still extremely thin, but no longer wearing the deathlike shadow mask she'd carried for so long. We drove home the next day and moved Erin into the bedroom that had served as a nursery when Ariel and Jocelyn were babies.

Meanwhile Zane moved out of our house into a local apartment for his sophomore year of college, and, with Jenna now away at school, the relative peacefulness I'd anticipated with just Jocelyn and Ariel in the house was displaced by the habitual wariness that accompanied having Erin's food rituals and trance-like television watching ever-present. Except for her trips to Walmart or the Dollar Store for binge food and her weekly therapy appointments, she was home most of the time. Perhaps because she had become accustomed to nurses and counselors being available around-the-clock, she was irritated if her immediate requests, whether for a particular food or time to talk, weren't met on her schedule. I reminded myself that she was dealing with both addiction and depression, and tried to be patient and compassionate, but the thought of having her with us for an extended period scared me. Her seclusion was a symptom of how depressed she felt, because she charmed others easily. I remember being at a shopping mall and meeting up with her after we had gone to different stores. She had befriended an older gentleman who was sitting on an outdoor bench, and he expressed how much he'd enjoyed talking with her.

During my afternoon breaks I would take her to the coffee shop, which was like a little haven for us to explore being people other than the struggling child and suffering mother. Getting out of the house helped us to relax with each other. I wasn't vigilant and she wasn't defensive. Even though she spoke about her therapy and the conflicting hope and despair she felt, I could listen to her more as a therapist and friend than as her mother. But it never seemed like enough. I also felt like the harried, distracted mother trying to get chores done while an insatiable toddler pulls at her skirt.

Though I questioned myself incessantly and often saw myself as uncaring and selfish, I saw a different image reflected by those who knew and loved me. In a birthday card Andrew's brother described me as having "strength of vision and undaunted compassion." My guilt and grief about Erin had been especially strong at the time, and I marveled that he saw me this way. I only saw myself through the dark glass of my frustration, impatience, and discouragement. He saw me as noble, while I saw myself as up against the wall, doing what I had to. What else could I have done — rejected her, committed suicide, been perpetually angry and depressed? There was no life-sustaining option other than to try to rise above and endure, and ultimately release myself and her. It was always easier to see where and how I had failed myself and her, than to see how well I managed. I saw the unloving parts of myself mirrored in Erin's eyes, and even when we had a soft and clear encounter, I still felt lacking.

Thanksgiving had just passed when I sat down to write our annual Christmas letter, a ritual I usually enjoyed and one that kicked me into the holiday spirit. I'd been putting it off because I couldn't portray our lives like a happy postcard list of successes and accomplishments, but I didn't want to sound like I was pleading for sympathy, either. As I looked back on the past year, I felt battle weary but not triumphant, the only triumph being in having survived.

Most of the letters we received each year listed the stellar accomplishments of gifted children, described family trips to

Europe and Hawaii, highlighted professional gains, and overall, painted an airbrushed picture of lives untainted by struggle and loss. Could it really be that easy for others?

When I finally put fingers to keyboard, I described happy and benign family happenings over the past year, while also including our sadness and fear for Erin. Despite the ongoing anguish about her, I expressed gratitude for a marriage that was loving and strong enough to sustain me, as well as for our wonderful children, with and without trophies. My life had room for it all, and I was relieved to express that without apology or pride.

17

CHAPTER

Jail

Suffering is the personalization we
bring to our difficulties.

JUDITH LASATER

"Erin's in jail."

Roger's voice was tense as he explained that she had been caught stealing food at a large grocery store in a city nearby. She was on probation for shoplifting at Walmart. She had enough control to drive and take care of her basic needs, so I still believed that, at age 20, she could be responsible for her behavior. Even as I felt the familiar rush of frustration with yet another infraction, I pictured her frail little body curled up on a cot, looking pathetic and lost in her baggy plaid shirt and green hat, her gaunt face drawn and hopeless. Alcoholics talk about hitting bottom. This must be it. Or is spending day after day with her head in a toilet bowl even lower?

At least she's safe, I tried to convince myself, while wondering how her body could survive the emotional impact of being locked in a lifeless, gray cell.

The next day I had just got home late from work on a cold, blustery night to a message that Erin was being released from jail at midnight "for good behavior." I couldn't imagine going back out in the blizzard, driving another 30 miles on winding unplowed country roads at midnight. I also had to pack and leave for a weekend training session at 6 the next morning. I called the jail and was told she could stay until 8 a.m., but they couldn't keep her any longer since she was legally an adult. I was more exhausted by the minute as weariness battled with guilt.

I called Roger, who was bowling with his Thursday night league, to see if he could go.

"Hell, no. I'm not going up there at midnight or at 8 a.m.!"

Andrew said he could rearrange his schedule to pick her up at 12:30 in the afternoon, so I called the officer at the jail and told him to let her know she could take a cab or wait for Andrew to come for her midday.

"There's a Dunkin' Donuts a block away, so she can wait for him there," he told me.

When I called back, he said that's where she would be.

After packing and eating a late dinner, I fell into bed, longing for sleep. Instead, the image of her tiny, frail body struggling through the cold and wind toward Dunkin' Donuts, and then huddled in the corner of a booth alone, haunted me throughout the night. Did she have money to buy a cup of tea? Would she be safe there? My mind ping-ponged between guilt, exhaustion, and justification. How could I leave her in that place when she didn't have to be there? Roger didn't seem to have any problem saying, "No way!" I wondered if he was insensitive and self-centered, or whether that was appropriate "tough love." I had conceded to his way of seeing the world for years, and this time it was convenient to use him as a reality check.

Yet other voices chided me, all those self-sacrificing mother messages that say, "Nothing is too much or too hard where your child is concerned."

But she put herself there. This is one of the consequences of her behavior! I argued back.

What should I do? On one hand I knew it wasn't up to me to rescue her from spending another night in the jail. She was lucky not to be there another week, as originally sentenced. And she could wait there if she chose to, in safety, until we were able to come. But my inner prosecutor poured on the guilt. The image of her clutching her second-hand coat around her body trying to keep out the wind and cold as she fought her way to the donut shop was a relentless slide show in my mind until I finally fell asleep, long after midnight.

A week later, when she was safely home and the storm of guilt had passed through me, we were sitting at the kitchen table, she with her mug of artificially sweetened herbal tea and me with my coffee.

"I want to go back to school," she said, "so that I can have some structure and direction in my life."

Maybe the harsh stint in jail a week ago had "scared her straight," and my heart took a cautious hopeful leap.

"Honey, that would be wonderful," I replied.

I tried not to dwell on how damaged her body must be. Maybe if she found some normalcy and success in college, she might recover something of a healthy life. Perhaps hope really does spring eternal.

Madonna or Martyr

You give but little when you give of
your possessions. It is when you
give of yourself that you truly give.

KAHLIL GIBRAN

One hot morning the following July, I took Erin and Jocie to the yearly arts festival in the town where Andrew and I have an office. Initially, I'd hesitated to ask Erin because I knew any lengthy outing would involve meals, but I thought she would enjoy the festival. She was delighted to be able to go.

After strolling for an hour along the street lined with pottery, photography, paintings, crafts, and jewelry exhibits, we were ready for lunch. Jocie and I picked out our food in short order, while Erin moved slowly from one booth to another, querying the vendors at length about the precise ingredients in their various offerings. Jocie and I stood holding our sandwiches and drinks, waiting for what seemed like hours for Erin to make up her mind. When she walked toward us at last, she was smiling, her bony arms carrying a white Styrofoam container of greens.

"There's a table over here," she called, her voice light and eager.

She's so happy to be here, I thought, battling the frustration I felt with her inability to eat anything but undressed salad after complaining about how hungry she was.

After finishing our lunches, we proceeded along the street. I had my eye out for a goldsmith from Rochester whose asymmetrical designs were among my favorites. Meanwhile, I watched for any clients who might pass by, and was relieved when Erin wandered to the other side of the street, too far away for anyone to notice that we were together. I was absorbed in examining some silver earrings when I felt a tap on my shoulder.

"Hi, Barb!"

I turned to face a slender, dark-haired 16-year-old client.

"Hi, Jen, how's it going?" I asked, a bit too brightly.

"Good," she replied.

I realized I was avoiding eye contact with her when she quickly added, "See you next week," and turned to follow her mother down the street.

Suddenly, I was aware of Erin at my side. How long had she been there?

Please don't let them notice her.

Despite Erin's hollowed cheeks and sharpened features, we looked like mother and daughter. Out of the corner of my eye, I saw Jen and her mother tip their heads together and then glance back at Erin.

They know, I told myself, the knot in my chest tightening.

My cover as Wise Woman in Control was blown.

I strode with my right arm around Jocie's waist while Erin walked happily along on my left, oblivious to my turmoil. Even though I counsel my clients to not let other people's responses control them, I was deeply ashamed that a client and her mother had seen me with my emaciated daughter. My insides tightened with guilt. What kind of mother am I, to be ashamed of my own daughter? My tidy, have-it-all-together professional persona had collided with my pain-spattered mother-world — Norman Rockwell painted over by Jackson Pollock.

By 4 p.m. I was ready to leave, and Erin agreed that she, too, had had her fill of heat and browsing. I sank into the hot car, immediately relieved at being sheltered from the possibility of being seen again. Erin sang along with the radio during the drive home. When I pulled up to the curb in front of her apartment, I reached across the gearshift to hug her.

"Thanks, Mom."

She squeezed me tightly before stepping out of the car with her tote bag and the gaily decorated ceramic bowl I'd bought her. Now that we were safely out of the public eye, I found myself wanting to replay that scene on the street, this time with my arm around Erin's bony little shoulders, pulling her close to my side.

Maybe I wasn't so bad, I consoled myself. *She had a good time. It's not like I abandoned her!*

The guilt loosened its grip on my heart a bit. Driving the last mile home, I felt as though I could breathe again.

My sense of peace was short-lived. A few days later, I was having lunch with Sally, a woman I'd known for 15 years. She had two daughters and a son, and over the years we'd shared many meals and heart-to-hearts. Though Sally and I no longer saw each other regularly, Erin remained close to her, often stopping by her house to chat. Sally seemed happy to offer my daughter her time and emotional support.

We sat across from one another in a booth at a local restaurant, the conversational buzz of the midday crowd humming around us.

"I know you've been spending time with Erin, and I really appreciate that," I began, conscious of feeling both gratitude and guilt that Erin needed another mother figure in her life. "She's lost even more weight, and now they've started her on some different medications. I keep hoping something will help, but she just gets worse and worse."

I looked into Sally's eyes, expecting her usual reassurance and empathy. Sally was quiet for a moment.

"Maybe it would help if you spent more blocks of time with her," she finally said. "She gets lonely a lot and needs to talk."

My body felt instantly heavy. I knew Sally meant well, but the thought of adding "blocks of time with Erin" to my to-do list made me feel exhausted, even suffocated. Mentally, I looked at my calendar for the next month; it seemed that every spare minute was already scheduled.

Don't you know how busy I am? Don't you understand that I have three other daughters and a stepson who also need my time and attention, as well as a marriage and career?

Why wasn't Sally, who had a habit of being exceedingly understanding and sympathetic, soothing me? I looked down at my half-eaten sandwich, my stomach tight and heart pounding.

"I know that Erin wants more from me," I murmured. "I just don't know if I can do it."

I hoped my defensiveness didn't come through in my voice. Sally was a caseworker, and in her free time, she championed the rights of the mentally ill. Self-sacrificing to the marrow, she routinely put the needs and wants of others before her own. I didn't want to be Sally, but I still wanted her approval. I left the restaurant feeling small and hard.

The next morning, still feeling remorseful and helpless, I remembered the power of asking for counsel from my wisest self by journaling. Sitting at the little table where I wrote and meditated in the early morning, I silently asked, "Should I be doing more for Erin?" I put my pen to paper and let the words flow:

> *Her life is hers to save. She wants to regress back to the womb with you because you were so safe, and it was a time of peace and joy for her. Her wounds came later. Your love for her is like food. She wants to binge on it, but can't hold it in because she doesn't believe she deserves it.*
>
> *To give unlimited quantities of time would not be helpful. She needs to learn to nourish herself on smaller amounts of food and love from you and hold that in . . . so it's like checking the cupboards and seeing that the food is there, even when it's not time to eat.*

I placed the pen down on the desk, read over the words, and felt a wave of relief wash over me. I wasn't neglecting Erin. I breathed deeply. Setting limits is a good thing. Closing my journal, I went downstairs to fix breakfast.

The journaling had helped me to see that my boundaries with Erin were supporting both of us. For a little while, at least, it helped me to simply "be" with her from that place the Buddhists call "non-attachment" — a state of accepting what is and letting go of outcomes. The writer Oriah Mountain Dreamer says that when we let go of wanting things to be a certain way, "we find ourselves truly at peace with what is often an unpredictable and sometimes messy human life." At that moment, my wise inner voice helped me embrace my own mess and see myself as just one mother doing her best to love a child whose life had gone dangerously off course — a life I had no power to restore.

Once in a while, I could do more than just feel a sense of acceptance — I could act from that calm, open-hearted place. I wished Sally could have witnessed the warm summer evening when I stopped by to visit Erin at the apartment I'd found for her at other end of town. The rooms were dark and small and the white clapboard was peeling, but she seemed content with it. A week after she moved in, I walked down to her apartment toting a plastic bag filled with assorted knick-knacks I thought she might like to use to decorate the place.

When she opened her rickety screen door I asked, "Would you like to take a walk with me?"

"I can't go yet," she replied. "I've been bingeing and I need to purge."

I tried gentle persuasion.

"Maybe you could use a walk as an opportunity to postpone purging," I suggested.

"I can't," she replied matter-of-factly. "Can you come back in ten minutes?"

"Sure," I found myself saying.

As I turned and headed down the sidewalk, I stepped lightly, surprised by the sense of softness and peace in my heart. For once, Erin hadn't been defensive, and I hadn't bitten back any frustration or disgust. I experienced a sense of wide-open acceptance that I'd never quite reached before. It was such a contrast to the familiar, painful tug-of-war between fear and love, and between self-doubt and self-preservation, that shadowed most of my interactions with her. *Thank you!* I whispered to myself, grateful for that moment of grace.

But only a few days later, in the safe haven of my office, my emotional roller coaster came crashing down from that lofty threshold.

"I was studying for my accounting exam and finally got to bed after midnight," began Marie, a middle-aged client I'd been seeing for several months. "Then Rachel called, crying and wanting to talk about her relationship with her boyfriend."

Rachel was her 20-year-old daughter.

"I was so tired, and she talked for over an hour," Marie went on. "When I told her that I had a big test the next day, she accused me of making school more important than her, and she hung up."

Marie looked up at me as if I were a magician who could untangle her dilemma with a wave of my wand. The anguish streaming from her pleading brown eyes told me that Rachel's attempts to make her mother feel guilty had worked. I felt my own anger rise.

I wanted Marie to be angry too; I wanted her to see that Rachel was being selfish and manipulative. But she wasn't finished.

"I felt so bad about it that I wanted to make it up to her," she told me. "She's crazy about Boyz II Men, so for her birthday I ordered a poster and all the CDs she didn't have yet. I thought she'd be thrilled. But when I gave them to her at the family party, she unrolled the poster and tore it into pieces and stormed out of the dining room."

Marie's eyes filled with tears.

I felt like wringing the ungrateful little brat's neck — not exactly the most professional response. For Rachel, nothing would ever be enough. For Marie, nothing was too much to do. My heart was beating faster as unwanted thoughts arose about how differently I dealt with Erin. What would Marie think of me with my daughter, the same age as hers, living in a dismal apartment and slowly starving to death? Steadying my voice, I suggested that Rachel was being unreasonable and reminded Marie of all the support she provided to her every day.

But Marie wasn't really listening. She began to talk about Peggy Claude-Pierre, a psychologist who ran the Montreux Clinic and who had recently published a book with a non-traditional approach to treating eating disorders. As Claude-Pierre explained on *Oprah* and other shows, she'd given up everything in her life to tend to her anorexic daughters 24 hours a day. She believed that their refusal to eat represented a fundamental lack of self-worth. To try to fill that void, she spoon-fed them bits of food, staying close to their sides and reminding them continuously of how precious and loved they were.

Listening to the story of this super-mother, I imagined myself shaping my life around feeding Erin like a helpless infant. Every fiber in my body screamed *NO!* Even though I knew this wasn't something I could do, I wondered if this place would be the answer for Erin. But how would we ever afford it? I struggled to keep my attention on Marie, who was expressing concern that Rachel was showing signs of an eating disorder. She wondered aloud whether she should try Claude-Pierre's approach on Rachel.

With those words, any remaining clinical objectivity was crushed like that ill-fated poster.

Barely maintaining a façade of calm, I asked: "Have you considered Rachel's responsibility to herself and the message you would be sending to her? And what about your own schooling?"

Marie appeared both puzzled and relieved, as if considering her own needs hadn't occurred to her.

"I just don't know. . . ." she said, her voice trailing off.

After she left, I closed the office door behind her and took a deep breath. My heart was still pounding with frustration and fear.

You matter too! I wanted to scream at Marie, but some shadowy woman in my head wagged her finger and said, "That's what good mothers do."

I remember one of my girls asking me, "How would you rather die — by burning to death or drowning?" (Sometimes I even got to choose death by either freezing or hanging.) It was the multiple choice from hell. That's how it felt now, to weigh the prospect of taking care of Erin and setting much of my current life aside, with no promise that that would "save" her, versus preserving my life while my daughter languished, hungering for my undivided attention. "None of the above" wasn't an option I saw.

Cactus Flower

If it were not for the divine hope
in us, our experiences would be more
than the human heart could digest.

ERNEST HOLMES

It was the early fall of 1997, and Erin had been home from Pittsburgh for only two months. She had steadily shed the 10 pounds gained there and regressed to her pre-hospitalization weight of 65 pounds. Once she reached her goal weight at a facility, insurance carriers would consider her ready to transition to outpatient treatment, even though it was the inpatient structure that kept her from binging, purging, and restricting. Dana (her current therapist at the local mental health clinic), Roger, and I agreed that there was no point sending her to another traditional medical setting. Instead, we decided to find a way to manage the cost of Remuda Ranch, a 12-step Christian program in Wickenburg, Arizona, devoted exclusively to treating teenagers and adults with eating disorders. Erin was excited about the idea of being in such a sunny climate, and the emphasis on Christianity appealed to her, as well. She spoke often about how her faith in Jesus sustained her, so I hoped that God and sunshine would join forces to create a healing that had eluded her thus far.

The challenge was coming up with the money to pay for the program, which could last many months depending on her progress or lack thereof. Medical Assistance had covered her last few hospitalizations and paid for her therapy, but Remuda Ranch wasn't eligible for public or private insurance reimbursement. Even Andrew, who had never withheld money, echoed my concern about spending tens of thousands of dollars with no assurance that the program would be able to help her. When I asked Roger, he said that he was unwilling to do more for the same reason.

However, Erin's enthusiasm about Remuda Ranch was in total contrast to the resistance she had expressed to prior hospitalizations, so, after much discussion, Andrew, Roger, and I came up with an arrangement that seemed fair to us all and called for investment from Erin as well. She agreed to using the amount left in her college account, with Roger and I each matching that—a sum that would cover several months in Arizona. We would be delighted to figure out how to pay for college later on if that meant she was healthy enough to go. Though no one said it out loud, this felt like her last chance at saving her life. She would leave shortly and be out there for her birthday in early October.

Like most 12-step programs, Remuda had a family component to treatment. They stopped just short of insisting that both parents come out for a week to participate in a class and family sessions with the patient's primary therapist. Roger had agreed to go for the week, which fell during his mid-semester break. Celia would accompany him. I was resisting the idea, partly due to the cost not only of flying and staying out there, but also the loss of a week's income. I wished that Andrew could come, but doubling the expenses along with the additional loss of income from our practice was out of the question.

Without my strongest ally and support, I was wary of family therapy that included Roger. I wanted to do what was best for Erin without setting myself up for more guilt and criticism — I did a good enough job of inflicting that on myself.

After wrestling with whether to go for weeks, I finally broke through the ambivalence by asking myself which decision I was likely to feel best about in 10 years. Which would reflect the person I would want to have been? That did it. I knew the impact of not earning income for that week would fade over time without major hardship, and that this was an opportunity for me to be there for Erin in a way that mattered to her. If I didn't go, I might regret it, and that regret would last a lifetime. I called Remuda to reserve my room for the Family Week at the end of October.

Once the decision was made, I was able to get on board with some excitement about seeing that part of the country, being able to visit with my sister who lived within several hours of Wickenburg, and, most importantly, feeling at peace with saying "Yes!" to Erin. I felt lightened and self-redeemed by agreeing to what she wanted from me.

Even so, I was still nervous about what Family Week would bring out. The underlying power struggle that continually resurfaced hadn't been resolved. I had laid down my weapon but didn't trust her enough to expose myself fully, not until several days before I was scheduled to leave and she called, her voice soft and full of pain, like an open wound.

"I'm so sorry for everything — for how I have hurt you all, and I can see why you have a hard time being around me."

Not only was my pistol on the ground, but with those words I felt the armor around my heart melt away. I had waited so long to hear this. A simple apology, and my anger dissolved. I wanted to reach across 10 states to enfold her. I was so grateful that her therapy at Remuda was empowering her to take some responsibility instead of wallowing in blaming others. She was working through the early stages of the 12 steps classic to Alcoholics Anonymous.

As the date to leave approached, I also began to see the potential to heal some of my unfinished business with Roger. This was about more than what might it open up between Erin and me. Strangely, I felt almost sisterly toward her, as if we were in this together, and I wanted to support her. It seemed like coming full circle back to her birth, and being there for her with Roger, but this time with more consciousness of my own power and worth.

I also realized that even though I would be without the major props in my life — Andrew, the girls, and my work — I would not be alone. And even though Andrew was my most powerful mirror, I had to remember that my reflection was only that. I exist as certainly without any mirror.

Just before I left, I had several dreams of near death, only one of which I remembered. We knew our house was going to burn down, so we were trying to get as many things as possible removed. As it got worse, I could see flames coming out of the walls and thought it was too dangerous to continue. I screamed for my mother (who, in real time, had been dead for 16 years) to stop working and come outside, but she wouldn't. I felt such helpless rage at her for being so stubborn to the point of risking her life. The flames finally died out, and she was there, covered with soot, standing on what remained of the concrete foundation. I was so relieved and amazed she had survived and briefly wondered if my panic had been unwarranted.

Even though my dream-mother put saving herself after doing what she thought she had to do, she survived. I wondered if that meant Erin would survive, or did it mean I would, no matter how much my life and personal shelters went up in flames?

My sister Brenda and her oldest daughter Sonja met me at the Phoenix airport, and the next morning I picked up my rental car and followed Brenda's van through the flat, dry saguaro and sagebrush landscape to Wickenburg. When we arrived at Remuda we visited together with Erin down by the horse corral, and by late afternoon Brenda and Sonja headed home. I settled into my room feeling the pang of missing Andrew on such a significant trip, and then took a walk at dusk around the surrounding suburbs of stucco, tiled roofs, and cactus gardens. I had my journal and several books for evening company and looked forward to the solitude. The Family Program started the following morning at 9.

During our morning introductions, I told the group that I had hope but no expectations for Erin. I was still grieving for the kind of future I'd wanted and anticipated for her, but I held onto the hope that she would survive, and beyond survival, live a life that felt meaningful to her. And that was enough for me. By lunchtime of the first day, it was clear that Erin had worked her magic, charming the parents of the patients in our group.

"She's such a dear, and so smart!" one of the other mothers exclaimed.

For the first time in years I basked in the glow of parental pride for my eldest child. Since most of the information about addiction and family patterns was familiar for me, I focused on paying attention to Erin, knowing I was there to learn more about how to be with her, rather than theories about cause and dysfunctional family dynamics.

In the early morning and evening I walked. One night, after getting back to the room, I wondered about Erin's attraction to the conservative Christian orientation of the place, so foreign to the kind of spirituality with which she'd been raised. Perhaps Erin related so strongly to the born-again version of Christ because she felt as though she carried the sins of the family — the compiled genetic baggage of her ancestry — and through the eating disorder she had nailed herself to the cross as the ultimate sacrifice. And at this time in her life, instead of feeling forsaken, she had faced all her fears of being abandoned and rejected, spoke of the sins she carried and contributed to, and felt free to resurrect into a new life with a new body. She would bear the internal stigmata of organ damage, bone loss, and a weakened heart. I wondered, could a new life also mean total regeneration and healing, reversing the effects of 10 years of physical devastation? I didn't want to focus on that, and instead thought that if she or I were to die today, at least we would have achieved a level of understanding and acceptance that would hopefully free our souls from manifesting these wounds again, displaying the wisdom and strength of well-healed scars.

With each day I felt more hopeful. Erin and I were enjoying a level of ease with each other that we hadn't had in years, and she seemed gratified at how well Roger and I were getting along. I expected this trend to continue, but when she came into the art therapy session on Wednesday afternoon where all the parents were already gathered, I knew from the set of her jaw and the way she stared straight ahead without looking at anyone that she was angry and closed-off once more. A quick glance at Roger confirmed that he, too, had noticed the shift. After the session, she walked out, not having spoken to anyone, before either of us could talk with her.

That evening I asked for guidance on how to keep my heart open to her during these periods of darkness, and wrote something in my journal that I hadn't consciously realized until I found myself writing the words:

She is here, you are here, to learn from each other. There is no sepa-ration. Whether or not she chooses to live has nothing to do with whether she has learned. The energy of your learning and Roger's learning has both released her and challenged her. She is now free to grow up, which she has never wanted to do. She has been the means for both of you to shed outworn ways of being, but unlike the Christ image you had earlier, she has not stepped in and claimed her own True Self. She doesn't trust it yet. She needs the fundamentalism because it gives her a certainty she doesn't have inside. Focus on the light at the heart of her faith. As she grows, she will internalize her father and her mother in a healthier, more balanced way, and then she can move into a more expanded and less sin-based, crucifixion-centered relationship with Christ. When Erin no longer experiences herself as nailed to the cross, she can step into the resurrected Christ. You have struggled so much yourself with shame and unworthiness, but you have always known your essential goodness. That is why you bristle at the hellfire and brimstone portrayals of God. Your horror at intentional cruelty is part of this knowing. It is as if you were watching one beloved child harm another. Would you eternally punish the one who was the aggressor? Of course not. All you would want would be for that child to become aware of where the real power lies, which is in the love of our true nature, and to "repent." The eating disorder is

*not Satan, but it is a separation from her True Self. Why would anyone,
in any way, separate from their True Self? Because we can't fully know
and appreciate the light unless we have experienced the darkness.*

The next morning, as I arranged my limp hair in front of the
small bathroom mirror, I blurted out, "I hate it!" Then I looked
right into the reflection of my eyes and felt an unexpected well
of compassion for how I'd spent so much of my life inspecting
my appearance for flaws and rarely measuring up. My heart ached
for all the years I'd abandoned myself through criticism and judgment — *I look fat in those pants, my hair is too straight and flat, my
chin is too soft and weak.* Did all my girls filter out their beauty and
zero in on their so-called imperfections, all readily reinforced by
the ubiquitous images of airbrushed and borderline-anorexic
models?

As Ward, our group facilitator, said in the Family Week
introduction, "Even Cindy Crawford doesn't look like Cindy
Crawford until the make-up artists and photographers have
worked on her for three hours!"

I wasn't ready to fondly embrace my flabby thighs as "the
aunties," like writer Anne Lamott has with hers, but I made a
small step out of incessant self-judgment by feeling the pain of
having been so unloving toward myself for so long. I felt a surge
of gratitude for Remuda, and what it was opening up in me.

20

CHAPTER

Faith and Family

Your wounds of love can only heal
when you can forgive this dream.

HAFIZ

We were aware when we chose Remuda Ranch for Erin that it followed a 12-step approach with a strong Christian orientation. Erin had been attending a local church and was enjoying and relating to the Sunday services. She had also charmed some of the older church ladies and basked in the grandmotherly concern she elicited from them. Even though we didn't attend a church ourselves, we were glad that she was finding more connection within the church community and great solace through her growing faith. She showed such spiritual sensitivity as a young child, and her involvement with Christianity gave her a medium that helped her believe that she mattered and was "saved," no matter what.

I had agreed to go to the worship service at Remuda the next morning with Erin because I knew that my being there would mean a lot to her. I met her outside the wooden swinging doors that opened into a large paneled room filled with folding chairs. The bright southwestern sun filled the room as the minister strode in, his head leading his body, hands clasped behind his back. He paced back and forth in front of the gathered parents, patients, and staff, a stiff smile on his face, as the stragglers settled into their chairs.

Relax! I admonished myself. *Give him a chance.*

But my arrogance detector was madly beeping in my ears. When he lamented the sorry state of human beings, sinners all, I tried to keep my usually transparent face as expressionless as possible. Erin wanted me here, and the least I could do was sit through this harangue. There was a large, painted wooden sign on the highway just south of our town that read, "The Fear of the Lord is the Beginning of Wisdom." I never liked that sign much, thinking that it missed the spirit of Christ's message. This sermon seemed to echo the essence of that sign.

I was checking my watch when he caught my drifting attention.

"Why, those New Age people think that everything is God! Imagine! That means that to them even this chair . . ." as he pointed to an empty seat ". . . is God!"

I didn't know what Erin might have said to some of the staff about my non-traditional spirituality, but suddenly this felt very personal. I had no way of knowing if I was even on his radar, but because I already felt like an outsider, I became acutely self-conscious.

"Why, you could even make yourself God!" he stated with a mocking tone that implied this was even more ridiculous, not to mention heretical, than worshipping the chair.

I don't think of myself as "New Age," and I haven't prayed to chairs or graven images of myself. But I could imagine how someone of his theology would see me that way. I took hold of Erin's hand, hoping she could see me through her own eyes. She smiled at me, and I smiled back, trying to hide my discomfort. It didn't matter whether she reconciled what she was hearing with what she knew about me. We were here, together, and that was what counted.

On the last night of the program, family members were invited to have dinner with the patients in the dining hall. As Erin and I talked while picking at a bland supper of broiled fish and steamed vegetables, she asked me to tell her more about my family history. I told her everything I could remember, which wasn't much, on both my mother's and father's sides. About my grandfather emigrating from Finland. That one of his brothers was a sword-swallower he hadn't heard from since he also left their native land. That because of my grandfather's socialist sympathies, he had considered going to Russia, but an older brother was already in the United States and had a factory job waiting for him. That he'd sent for my grandmother, who was, at 29, becoming unmarriageable for those days and ready to leave the childhood home where her father was an angry alcoholic. Though she missed her mother and sisters terribly and sent boxes of clothing to them every few months, she returned to Finland only once when I was a child. My mother was born five years after my grandparents married, an only child because, according to my grandmother, my grandfather didn't want the expense of more children.

I told Erin about how I spoke Finnish before English because my mother left me in Granny's care so that she could resume teaching and save the money my parents would need to buy a house. And about how I fell down a long flight of stairs when I was three. My father, who had been lying on the couch immobilized by sciatic pain, jumped up and carried me to the kitchen sink to rinse off my bleeding forehead before he and my mother took me to the hospital for stitches.

I knew even less about my father's family — mostly that he'd had nothing nice to say about his flaky, disorganized mother and had just begun to develop a rich, adult relationship with his father when he died of renal failure before my parents were married. My father's parents had divorced after 25 years of marriage. My grandmother went on to survive three more husbands and, because she lived in Florida, we saw her at most once a year. As a little girl I loved snuggling up beside her on the couch and hearing stories about my Aunt Jean, my father's next older sister, who was the creative mischief-maker of the three of them. Still a delightful eccentric at 85, Jean has conversations with her cat and dog who, it appears, understand her perfectly.

I told Erin about how I felt as a child — so awkward and wanting to be perfect in order to be loved, as well as the sweet memories of riding with my father on Saturday mornings as he replenished the gin supply for his daily martini and drove me to my art classes at the Albright Knox Art Gallery. Erin's eyes were soft and smiling, and I felt like we were in a sacred bubble, immune to the fluorescent lights, surrounding chatter, and clatter of dishes and silverware. After we finished eating, we stood outside the dining hall doors, my arms around her shoulders and hers around my waist. I didn't want to leave her. I didn't want to lose her. She was nesting in the center of my heart again, as years of mutual hurt, anger, and disappointment evaporated into the cool evening air.

I had her back, resurrected in my heart yet still fragile in the world, a tiny bird with a broken wing resting in my palm. For so long it had been a relief to have her far away, presumably safe, so I could live my life without the interference and static of her moods and behaviors. But now I wanted to hold her close, to stay connected and protect her however I could from the demon disorder. Maybe if I loved her enough, and she felt it enough, she would have the strength to fight the disease in those inevitable low moments. There had been a time when the thought of her dying would seep through the membrane of my mind. When that happened, I believed that I had already lost her to such an extent that much of my grief would be done. Taking her in like this meant I could lose her again. But even if my injured bird would never fly, the delicate weight of her warm body was imprinted on my heart.

Why did it have to be so hard for her? I would listen to clients' stories and read about others whose life circumstances had been far more abusive, negligent, and unsupportive. If all these factors are causal, then she shouldn't be this way. No one ever mentioned any fallout from the Sydenham's chorea, and my lightbulb moment in the espresso shop had faded into the background behind her ongoing behaviors and the appearance of choice and control. She was like my mother's English bone china tea cups, so delicate and fragile that they were nearly transparent — too fine to put in the dishwasher, needing to be gently washed and dried by hand, and then carefully placed back in the china cabinet behind glass doors. I, on the other hand, felt like a piece of everyday crockery with chips along the rim and hairline cracks in the glaze, still serviceable and microwave safe.

The day before we had that dinner together, I'd given Erin a purple T-shirt with whimsical dancing desert creatures, which I'd bought at a local gift shop. It reminded me of the playful animals and sprites she drew and of the giggling little girl she'd been, and whom I occasionally still glimpsed in light moments.

"I don't want it!" she declared inexplicably, when I gave her the tissue-wrapped offering, her face a hard angry mask.

I swallowed my disappointment and left it with her anyway, suggesting she give it to Sonja the next time Brenda came for a visit. It was too small for an adult or any of her sisters.

During the farewell gathering for Family Week, many of the parents and other patients commented on my strength and caring. Those words were like rain falling on hard, dry ground, most of it washing away because the surface wasn't soft enough to absorb what it needed most. I was so aware of holding part of myself back, keeping one foot on the island of an identity that could, at times, pretend she wasn't there.

I left Arizona appreciating a landscape that I had expected would be too dry and brown for me to enjoy. Depending on the time of day, the mountains edging the horizon were shades of copper to earthy mauve, the ancient majestic saguaro cacti holding court over the choya, ocotillo, and palo verde. Like Erin, they clung to life with little nourishment, explosive pink and yellow flowers tucked along prickly spines, beauty bursting out of barrenness.

Roller Coaster

If you are willing to surrender
to love rather than trying to control
it, love teaches you who you are.

GANGAJI

When I called Erin several days after arriving home, she said she couldn't imagine handling life on her own. Even the structured housing program provided by the transitional living facility called Chandler seemed like too much for her. It was designed to help those leaving the program to transition to more independent living and self-responsibility.

"Just take things one day at a time," I reminded her, hoping I sounded more confident in her ability to deal with the coming challenges than I felt.

I felt like the caring coach who encourages the team klutz to "Go out there and show them what you've got!" I wanted her to draw strength from my belief in her capacity to cope, despite how tenuous that felt to me. I clung to the idea that there was still a seed of wholeness in her that was taking root, and that my heartening words didn't betray the despair in my stomach when she sounded so fragile and afraid.

I had been home for a week when I listened to Erin's voice on the answering machine: "I'm sorry I told you I didn't like the shirt. It wasn't the shirt. I was pushing you from me the way I have for years, and I'm sorry. I'll wear the shirt. I really do like it." My roller coaster of hope edged up the track a bit. I breathed deeply, letting some of the tension go that I didn't even realize I was carrying.

Erin lived at the transitional placement in Chandler more than three months. Although her counselors didn't say it, when I spoke with them I heard between the lines of their carefully chosen words that Erin might not make it. Images of her as she was when she left for Remuda, skeletal and cadaverous, flooded my mind. I didn't want to see her like that again. I didn't want to watch her marching toward death, one binge and purge at a time, or witness her grilling waitresses about whether there was a trace of cheese or croutons in a salad, and then chewing her lettuce and carrot shreds slowly, eyes glazed, as if there were some non-fat food nirvana to which she was temporarily transported. I had believed, for a short time, that all of this could be in the past.

When one of her therapists asked about any family history of mental illness, I told her that Roger's brother had been diagnosed with bipolar illness, and I suspected her father's mood swings might be a milder version of that.

"We're trying to sort out how much Erin is thought-disordered, possibly even with some psychotic symptoms, and how these may have driven and supported the eating disorder," the therapist continued. "We're focusing on an underlying Obsessive Compulsive Anxiety Disorder and plan to treat that more aggressively with medication."

She paused, and then continued with a tentative tone: "Would you be upset if we classified her as seriously mentally ill in order to access more assistance?"

She had no idea how small this felt in the big picture of Erin's struggle. It was even a relief — a diagnosis that was independent of what I could have or should have done. Anything that might help her have more quality of life and tap into available services sounded like a good idea.

How sad that I'm not more sad, I thought.

I felt detached and clinical, as if I were discussing a client instead of my own daughter, the geographical space between us encouraging an emotional distance that was both comforting and disturbing. I wore the hat of the professional when I spoke with the staff about diagnoses, my fragile, wounded motherhood taking cover beneath a calm, clinical assessment that put even emotional disturbance into a neatly labeled box that was sealed tight.

"I miss you all so much," Erin began when she called in February from Chandler. "I know I thought I wanted to be here in the sun, but it's so far and it's already hot. I don't think I could stand it in the summer. I need to find somewhere else where I can get help with my OCD."

Was she asking me to find such a place? If so, I didn't feel up to the task. I wanted her to take care of herself, though I knew that the very fact that she had to have such a setting meant she couldn't handle that. I still wasn't ready to face her dependency

— it seemed so contradictory to the iron-fisted control she wielded around food. I wanted to reach out and hold her and protect her, but I didn't want her back home unless I knew the old food behaviors and rituals weren't coming with her.

But what I wanted didn't matter. She was coming home. I hadn't seen her since last fall in Arizona, and now it was February. I should be thrilled to know that the daughter I hadn't seen in four months was coming home, but I was neither happy nor unhappy, another obvious indicator of how far from normal we were. "I'm never going back to where I was before," she assured me, and I wanted to believe her. How wonderful if that were true. Where was her power and spirit now? Who was she? Did her fundamentalist Christian friends know her better than I did? I felt my wall begin to rise, behind which I watched every word and tried to prevent any unguarded emotion from escaping the landmine-loaded field of her perception. She said she'd changed, but was it true? Where was the sweet unburdened connection we felt after our last supper at Remuda?

Every day I awakened to dread creeping into my stomach with the dawn as I worried about having her in the house again. I could relax when she was safely tucked away, in someone else's care. It was the end of February, and again, I looked within myself and found the answer:

Just be there and love her without pressure and without fear. Let her know she matters to you and to the world. She feels very useless right now, without purpose and without strength of will to battle the disease. Few who could possibly understand have ever survived. Her body has to learn how to hold her feelings. Life feels like too much for her, and she needs you to stay close right now.

Though my daily routines pushed the awareness that Erin would be home in two days to the back of my mind, I awakened in the middle of the night with images of her wasting away. Even Andrew's gentle snoring wasn't enough to comfort me. And then, in the soft, defenseless place of semi-consciousness, protective love gushed out of my heart, flooding the landscape of remembered betrayals, disappointments, and lost dreams and washing away any angry debris. I wasn't worried about her stealing food or money, but only about whether she would completely succumb to the disease. Even though I sometimes thought, with pain in my heart, that death would finally bring relief to her poor ravaged body, I realized I would swim through the graveyard mud to save her. I just wanted her to claim some of the life she had never lived.

At this point Erin was 21, and living with us or her father on a long-term basis was out of the question. She wanted to be in her own space, and neither one of us wanted to repeat the watchdog role that seemed inevitable when she was living in one of our homes and that only interfered with being with her as lovingly as possible. So before she returned from Chandler, I checked out apartments in town that she could afford with her Social Security Disability income and some help from us. I found a place less than a mile away from our house that seemed adequate, and though the white clapboard exterior was peeling, I imagined how it could be cozied up inside with the furniture her father and I had for her, and, of course, her own drawings on the wall.

Erin moved into the apartment shortly after getting home, in early March 1998. The therapists at Chandler had arranged for local casework services, and she'd be seen by Dana, whom I considered the best therapist at the local clinic. After Erin got settled in, she started working a few hours in the evenings at a local video rental store. It was too late in the spring semester for her to attend classes at the university, but she hoped to take at least one course at a time during the summer and continue in the fall.

It had been a cold, gray Saturday in early April, and I was weary from all the weekend household chores by the time Andrew and I sat down after dinner to start watching a movie. I didn't want to take care of anyone or anything for the few hours before going to bed. Just as I'd curled myself against Andrew on the sofa, the front door opened and Erin walked in. My disappointment at having our brief respite interrupted dissolved into aching sadness as I watched her slide her bulky teal and red plaid winter coat off fleshless shoulders.

"Can I talk to you alone?" she asked, tears filling her large green eyes.

She followed me into the kitchen/family room area, away from the television, and we sat down together on the loveseat.

"I got so panicky I had to leave my job today." Erin had started working two weeks earlier as a part-time clerk at a video rental store. "I know I should be doing something with my life, with my art, but I'm so scared. I can't handle going to classes. I think I'll mess up, and I won't find the place to register or the classroom."

Her life sounded like one of the anxiety dreams I used to have, in which I couldn't find my way and I was already 20 minutes late for the final exam. I always woke up, relieved to find that I was dreaming, while she longed to go to sleep and forget the nightmare of her daily life. I put my arm around her shoulders, feeling the sharpness of unbuffered bone. I wanted to tell her she could handle school, that she was brighter than most of the students there, and that her fears were the normal anxiety we all have from time to time. But I didn't believe it, either. Holding her close was the only reassurance I had to offer. As she rested her head on my shoulder, I could see her scalp where she had pulled her hair back with a clip. Even her hair was getting thinner.

After sitting quietly for a short while, she said, "I'm hungry."

"I have some leftover pea soup in the refrigerator," I offered.

My thick homemade split pea soup had always been one of her favorite foods.

"I can fix it myself," she said, so I left her alone in the kitchen and went back into the living room to watch the movie.

I heard the water running and knew she was diluting her soup, but I didn't get up to check.

Let go! I reminded myself.

She brought her microwaved mug of watery soup into the living room and curled up next to me on the couch, nesting like a frail wounded bird against my side. She lifted one small teaspoonful at a time to her mouth, sighing contentedly as the warm soup reached her shrunken stomach. Liquid love snuck past the demon disease, temporarily displaced by a mother's embrace. I held her close for the rest of the movie.

As she put on her coat to leave, I said, "I don't want to lose you."

"I don't want to lose you, either," she replied.

Before the week was out, Erin had quit the job. Dana, her therapist, and Jill, her caseworker, arranged for her to attend a partial hospitalization program three days a week. The agency provided transportation to "Partial," as it was called, so all Erin had to do was pack a lunch for herself. She loved it. Within the first week she had charmed the staff with her brightness and insight, and, instead of feeling like a failure, she had found a group in which struggling to manage life was the norm. I was relieved that she had some structure to her days — something to look forward to besides soap operas and ritual bingeing and purging.

One evening in mid-May, Erin called to tell me that she was doing better.

"I had an ice cream cone when I went miniature golfing with a friend, and I kept it down," she said proudly.

"That's great, honey," I replied, and then we chatted about her week at Partial and plans for the weekend.

The next morning I wrote in my journal:

I hear that, but my heart doesn't leap, and my mind doesn't start thinking, "Maybe this time she can do it." There's actually very little hope in this void of expectation. She has long ceased to be the daughter I could celebrate and enjoy. I watch her sisters unfold into the future, ever stronger, more beautiful, meeting the challenges and joys of life with energy. Even when the violent winds of teen life blow them down, like well-rooted trees they slowly right and reach for the sun again. Erin seems to have never gotten her roots into the soil. Being alive was too much for her. Yet in some ways I marvel at her strength to keep going in her condition with the uncertainties and limitations that are now hers forever.

A week later, I reflected further:

This has been a fairy-tale transformation turned inside out and upside down — happy beginning to sad, lingering end. And what is the moral of the story? So many possibilities have gone through my mind and shadowed my life over the past 10 years — her father's temper, having to share me with her sisters, my own preoccupation with weight, my inadequate sense of self. I'm so ready to take it all on as mine, but I know I was a good mother. If all children took their parent's neuroses and internalized and magnified them to the extent Erin did, the world would fall apart.

And then, less than a month later, I got a call that Erin was back in the local hospital behavioral science unit (BSU) for depression and because her white blood cell count was so low. I called the hospital to speak with her, but she was out for a walk.

"We just realized that she has been bingeing and purging every night, and she is down to 66 pounds," the nurse told me.

When I finally talked with Erin an hour later, she said she was overwhelmed at the thought of having to make a life for herself.

Though my words were blunt, my voice was gentle: "Wouldn't it be easier going to bed at night knowing you had done something to contribute to the world than starving through the day waiting for a chance to binge and purge? Instead of thinking in terms of getting rid of the disorder, why not accept that it will always be there to some extent and focus on ways to live a meaningful life around it?"

Something else had to matter, or she would never recover at all, and I couldn't let her see how hopeless I felt, too. Sometimes I suspected I was the only ballast that kept her from floating away completely, and I was weary from keeping her afloat yet also within reach.

"I'll be over tomorrow after work," I promised.

The next day, when I sat down on her bed, the afternoon sun brightened the room in the BSU she had to herself. The bed reminded me of the maple headboard I had as a child, the usual metal hospital bed replaced with a homey touch of normalcy behind locked metal doors.

"Thanks for coming, Mom."

I took her hands in mine. She had inherited my bone structure, now in miniature, and her hands, so cool and barely fleshed, looked like ghostly versions of my own. I choked down the sob that wanted to erupt from the ever-present well of sorrow in my chest, hoping she could absorb the love pulsing through my strong, solid hands, and tried not to feel the sadness that was joined to it. How could this losing her — that had gone on for so long — still be so hard?

"I didn't binge yesterday, and I'm trying not to today. I know I could get away with it here," she said, lifting her head from gazing at our joined hands.

"That's wonderful, honey," I replied, looking into her lovely green eyes, so large in her hollowed face.

"I'm so afraid I'll never be better, but if I did get well, I wouldn't know how to live a life without it. I just want to die. And I feel terrible saying that to you, my mother. I don't know how you've been able to stand watching me do this."

The tightness in my throat released with the truth we both knew and that hadn't been spoken before. I had let go of any expectations that she would recover a long time ago. She didn't have to pretend that she wanted to be saved, and I didn't have to pretend that I could save her. All I had was the occasional, barely flickering hope that she could salvage something that resembled a life out of the ruins of the past 10 years.

"I hate being 21, with so many more years to live!"

Her sadness and despair were deeper than anything I had known, while she feared having a future and identified with the disease that had stolen it from her.

"I don't enjoy anything," she continued. "Starving gives me such a driving need that bingeing satisfies like nothing else can. For a moment I'm fulfilled. I let myself have a need and satisfy it. That's the only place in my life that it's okay."

"But what about your artwork, and being with other people?"

I pleaded for her to see her gifts as I did. To feel them. Her eyes filled with tears.

"I love people," she admitted. And she was right. Whether it was in Alcoholics Anonymous meetings, which she attended because of the addictive pull of the eating disorder, or church, or her partial hospitalization program, Erin made friends wherever she met.

We talked about finding a living situation that would be more communal, the options in the area, and the insecurities that kept her from going to college. And then visiting hours were over. As I stood up to leave, I tried to see the face of the beautiful young woman she could have been.

Could that still be? I wanted to wonder, but couldn't let my mind go there.

We walked slowly down the hall to the locked doors through which only I could pass, and said goodbye.

As I drove home, I lingered with the depth of her despair that went beyond what I had ever known. I may have been down and hopeless, and even entertained thoughts of dying, but my despondency stemmed from my grief, profound disappointment, and sense of having failed her, and not because I couldn't imagine putting one foot in front of the other. It was more a question of whether I felt life was worth the effort, an effort I'd always known I was capable of making. Like rocking my crying baby back to sleep in the middle of the night or meeting with clients when I wanted to curl up in a chair and be nurtured myself, I did what had to be done — one step at a time. But she could barely lift her own weight.

Love and Resignation

The only thing that makes life possible
is permanent, intolerable uncertainty;
not knowing what comes next.

URSULA K. LE GUIN

Several weeks later, when Erin was back in her apartment and looking more skeletal than ever, I decided to visit her on a sunny Saturday morning on the way home from walking to the post office. Her door was open, so I knocked and walked in. She stepped out of the bathroom and stuffed two Dunkin' Donuts boxes into her garbage container. She didn't say anything, and neither did I. I sat down on the nubbly brown couch covered by the crocheted rainbow afghan her grandmother made, and she sat down next to me. Phoebe the cat rolled and purred at my feet as I bent over to scratch her copper-colored head and rub her white belly.

"How often are you purging?" I asked.

"Just once this morning," she answered, "and I didn't last night."

She knew that I wondered if she kept down the dinner she had eaten with us yesterday.

"Can I come home with you and spend some time at the house?" she asked. "I don't have anything to do today."

I felt the weight of the day hanging on her.

"Of course, honey," I replied, while thinking that she needed something else to look forward to, as well. "Why don't you call someone to see about getting together tonight, or start reading a new book?"

Even that seemed like more than she could handle at the moment. We started walking toward home, and when we passed through the middle of town along Main Street, I was aware of how much less I cared what passersby may have thought. I felt lighter and more connected to her without that suspected criticism from others hovering like a dark cloud over my head.

"I got information on a few more hospitals from the National Eating Disorder Association yesterday. You could call them both this afternoon from the house," I suggested.

"I don't know. . . ."

A part of her drifted off with her voice, and we walked without talking the rest of the way.

She sat at the kitchen table leafing through magazines as I baked brownies for dessert. Then she helped me take the laundry off the clothesline, and we headed to the car wash. I was conscious of leaving her alone in the car as I aimed the hot soapy power spray at the windshield. When I moved around the trunk with the foaming brush, I saw her look back at me and then reach for my wallet where I had left it on top of the cup holders. I stopped scrubbing and looked into her eyes. She pulled her hand back into her lap. I finished washing, rinsing, and waxing, more conscious of the heavy sadness in my heart than the job at hand. No anger, no railing at her in my head, no righteous indignation — just sad that she could do that and still be so connected to me. I knew it wasn't personal — that it was just about what she could get away with.

I got back in the car, rolling down the windows as we pulled out of the concrete stall.

"I just wanted to see what was in there," she said.

I was silent. The wipers were clearing the last of the rinse water off the windshield, but nothing she said or I might have replied could clear the film of sadness that had settled on my heart. In the past I would have cried, "How could you do that!" hoping that guilt about stealing from her own mother would be enough impetus for her to control her behavior. I *wanted* her to see my anger and disappointment. After spending my life trying to please, and especially trying to avoid letting anyone else down, I still couldn't imagine how that wasn't enough motivation. But even mother-guilt paled in the face of her addiction-driven fear, and I felt only heart-wrenching resignation in the face of what neither of us could change. She knew that I knew she was lying, and we both knew she couldn't help herself.

As I pulled the car up in front of her apartment, she said, "I'm sorry."

I stroked the back of her head.

"I love you, honey. Please take care of yourself tonight," I said, which was my code for, "Don't binge and purge."

"I'll try," she said, as I reached across the gearshift to hug her.

She got out of the car and walked slowly to her door. I drove home, my mind still parked in the image of her large eyes pleading for the love I could never withdraw. When she left after dinner the night before, Andrew said, "I never know if this will be the last time I see her."

Though I wished the times we spent together would have some hint of normalcy, even when she smiled sweetly, the image of a Halloween house of horrors skull jumped into my mind the way it pops out in a spook house from a dark corner.

Late one afternoon when we were in the kitchen working on a family dinner together, I asked, "What's your agreement with Dana about weight and staying safe?"

Erin stood over the sink, snapping off the bud ends of green beans.

"I actually lost weight when I was in the hospital, so being there doesn't help, and Dana forgot to weigh us at the eating disorder group last week."

I felt a rise of anger with Dana because when I'd spoken with her the week before, she said, "I think Erin looks better, and she seems less depressed and has been expressing some hope and investment in life."

So she'll die happier instead of sadder! I wanted to say.

Dana's lack of emotion, at least with me, threw my horror at Erin's appearance into bold relief. Even though Erin was my daughter, Dana's calmness made my reactions feel distorted and extreme.

Yet when a friend who had seen Erin walking down Main Street said, "I don't know how you do it!" I felt validated and soothed by her empathy and acknowledgment of how bad it really was. I'd been "doing it" for so long that I didn't think of it as an accomplishment. After all, what choice did I have? Yet even Andrew, who'd been my greatest support and comforter, couldn't completely understand. We were stopped at the traffic light in the center of town when Erin walked by, and he said, "I think about what that would be like if it were Zane, almost like he and I were living in two different worlds that I couldn't bridge."

Meanwhile, as Erin put the trimmed beans in the steamer basket, she admitted her persistent weight loss was slow suicide: "I'm too scared to get healthy, and I don't think I can ever live up to what everyone seems to think I can do. Everyone keeps telling me how talented and bright I am. I can't handle even *thinking* about doing something. I can't live up to that!"

I knew that being at Partial was so helpful because most of the people there were much lower functioning than she. They probably never had the dreams for themselves or expectations from others that she'd lived with, and so, around them her comparing mind could relax, secure that, at least there, she wasn't a failure.

We worked quietly for a few minutes, and then she continued, "By the way, *Dateline* did an exposé on Peggy Claude-Pierre and the Montreaux Clinic, and they don't cure everyone like they said."

Even though we'd never seriously considered or discussed the possibility, I'd been feeling guilty about not calling just to check on whether Montreaux was an option for Erin. I felt instantly relieved. Erin continued, saying that reporters had uncovered practices that are illegal, such as force-feeding and not allowing people to leave. Though I was saddened that there wasn't a miracle cure, I was relieved that I hadn't failed my daughter by not getting her there somehow.

On July 29, 1998, after nine years of struggle, I wrote in my journal:

> *One of the things I have learned is that I can live with this, with the loss, the fear, the uncertainty. All of that has softened me through the humbling process of powerlessness and sadness that wash up on the*

shores of my daily life like the ebb and flow of the tides. . . . How can she hate herself so much to punish her body this way? I'm reminded of newspaper stories about psychotic abusive mothers tying up and starving their children. Yet here the victim and abuser are one. We can't rescue the victim and give her a chance at life because she is inexorably bound to her tormentor. She will go home and cruelly tease her body with the promise and hope of fullness, gorging on pretzels or animal crackers, perhaps assisted in their passage by a stick of butter, only to make herself purge it all, to deny any lasting satisfaction, like the sadistic parent throwing the food in the garbage as the starving child is forced to watch.

The day following that journal entry, I called Dana, but she wasn't in. I began wondering whether the professionals had given up on Erin and were planning to "let" her die. After all, nothing anyone tried so far had worked to break her free.

False Alarm

Courage is the ability to cultivate
a relationship with the unknown.

DAVID WHYTE

Several weeks later, on a warm, breezy mid-August morning, I
was relieved when my 11 a.m. client canceled, giving me time
to photocopy progress notes in response to a subpoena. I had
never appeared in court, and I was already anxious about being
called to testify in a custody hearing for a former client. I was
startled to hear a knock on the office door, which rarely happened unless someone was coming for a session.

Erin's case manager, Joanne, stood on the top step and
asked, "Can I talk with you privately?"

I motioned for her to step in and closed the door.

"I'm so worried about Erin. She didn't show up at Partial this morning, and the screen door to her apartment is locked."

An unbidden image appeared in my mind's eye, and I shared it with Joanne: "What if she's lying on that dingy brown shag carpet in her apartment, unconscious or dead?"

Joanne said, "That's what I'm afraid of, too."

"We have to call 911!" I declared.

"I *am* 911," she replied, "but I don't have the authority to break in."

We decided to call the police and have them meet Joanne at Erin's apartment. I had a client due to arrive shortly who was traveling a great distance to see me, but I assured Joanne I would answer the phone, which I don't normally do during a session. I tried to distract myself by continuing the tedious task that had been interrupted, but my hands were shaking as I placed one page after another on the tabletop copier. I'd been bracing for a moment like this for years, even wishing at times for the agony to be over for her, but I wasn't as ready as I'd thought.

Fifteen long minutes later the office phone rang, and I heard Joanne's voice: "We got in, but Erin wasn't there. I'm going to look for her around town, and if I find her, I'll hospitalize her myself."

She'd spent time with Erin over the past few days and knew how terrible she looked, that her weight was down to 60 pounds, and that her white blood cell count was also dangerously low. I was furious with Dana. Why wasn't she doing something? I called her office, and after being told by the receptionist that Dana was out of town at a conference, I left a heated message.

"You haven't returned my calls. She looks like death! I need you to call me as soon as you get back!"

Within the next hour Joanne called to say that Erin had arrived at Partial.

"The doctor is giving her one week to get her act together, or else she goes inpatient, whether she wants to or not."

I wanted to scream at the entire treatment team, *But she could be dead in a week!*

That evening I wanted to get out for a walk as soon as my sessions were over to release some of the nervous energy I'd had to contain all afternoon in order to sit with my clients. I was nearly out the door when the telephone rang.

Erin's voice was strong and upbeat: "I just wanted to say hi. I've had such a good day."

Have I just been dropped into the Twilight Zone?

I told her about the thought-to-be-crisis that morning.

"I had no idea about all that," she told me. "I was late getting to the bus for Partial, but someone gave me a ride."

She also explained that her rickety screen door tended to stick but hadn't been locked.

"Joanne told me what the doctor said," I said. "You have to start taking care of yourself if you don't want to go into the hospital. Not being depressed isn't enough."

"I know," she replied, without the defensiveness I expected.

"Honey, I love you," I said, pleading for her to understand that she mattered. "I was terrified about you this morning. I don't want that false alarm to come true."

"Thank you . . ." Her voice seemed to drift off. "I love you so much, Mom."

The following Monday Erin called back, but this time her tone was righteous and challenging.

"I need your work number in Corning to give Dana. She wants to set up a meeting with you, me, and Joanne because Joanne violated confidentiality when she came to you the other day."

"We were afraid you were lying there dead!" I was stunned that she couldn't acknowledge how real that possibility seemed to anyone who cared about her.

"It's my life, and no one else has the right to control it!" she said, planting her self firmly on the ground with what little weight she had.

"And when someone appears to be in danger, confidentiality isn't the point anymore," I asserted. "I'm also angry with Dana for not calling me back herself."

Her tone softened. "I don't know how you do it, seeing me look like this."

Her momentary awareness and empathy surprised me more than her usual apparent denial. I didn't know why, for a brief moment, she stepped out of her distorted and self-justifying mode and saw the situation through my eyes, but I was grateful.

Later that evening Jenna and I were walking down Main Street. Erin was getting into Celia's red Highlander with two Styrofoam to-go containers from the restaurant we were passing when she spotted us.

"Will you walk me home?" she asked. "I'm eating real food now. Something inside shifted after talking with Andy on Sunday, and I can feel God's help in beginning to change. I've gained six pounds since Friday."

"That's great, honey," I replied, trying not to sound hollow.

Jenna and I walked with her the half-mile to her apartment. After we left her there, Jenna said, "How many times has she said she is getting better?" This was after Erin had told us two days before that she couldn't get out of bed without lifting her legs with her hands, and that when she fell backward the other day, she didn't have the strength to get up. So that's why she was eating a little more! Did she think she could bargain with her body forever? If you give me some strength, I'll repay you with some food. But just enough to get by. Did she think her body was as easily deceived as her mind?

Over Labor Day weekend, I wrote:

Her bare bones are taking me down to my bare bones. Keeping my heart open doesn't mean I experience joy. Keeping my heart open means I don't cover myself with the different guises that fear can take — self-pity, self-justification, and self-defense.

Erin sounded strong and upbeat when I answered the phone a few days after her 22nd birthday.

"I just called to see how you're doing," she said.

"I'm fine, honey, just busy as usual. How are you?" I asked.

"I'm having trouble with gaining weight," she replied. "Three-and-a-half pounds. And I've been thinking about how I'm just taking and not giving anything with my life, and that maybe I would feel more invested in life if I were contributing something."

I felt hope — something that had eluded me for so long — rise up slowly within me. Having her say she wanted to be more invested in life in a long-term way — not just her daily routines of going to the day program and waiting for the magic hour when she permitted herself the gratification of her ritual big binge. Maybe this was the answer, the key that would unlock the door and finally free her to live more engaged in the world than in that obsessive little cage that circumscribed what she let in and out.

"I spoke with the minister at the Roseville church," she continued, "and he said I could visit shut-ins and help them with chores around the house and give them some company. I'm thinking of Tuesdays, since I don't go to Partial."

Her voice was so sweet and clear that my mind settled blissfully into the possibility that she might find some meaning and purpose in this simple but profound way. Her spirits lifted whenever she spent time with others, and being of service to others was an additional benefit. Several Tuesdays came and went because she didn't feel up to going, and I stopped asking her about it. My hope once again receded back to the dormant place it had occupied for years.

It was August 1, the anniversary of my mother's death. As I thought about her, I felt soothed as I imagined that she would be there to help Erin as she crossed over. The thought that Erin would likely die before long had been playing at my mind for a while and even seemed inevitable if she continued to lose weight. As painful as it was to think of her dying, it was almost more painful to envision her continuing as she was. She had entered this world with all the talent I longed for and couldn't own in myself, and all the fear, self-doubt, and deep shame that weighed me down had totally crippled her. She was the embodiment of the light and the shadow, and Heaven and Hell warred within her.

I had come far enough to know that it wasn't my fault she couldn't handle all that she contained, and I chose to believe that she would, at some time, accomplish what she seemed to have failed to do in this lifetime. My connection to her is eternal, and I took comfort in that.

24

CHAPTER

Sam

I want to know
if you can sit with pain,
mine or your own,
without moving
to hide it or fade it or fix it.

ORIAH MOUNTAIN DREAMER

I first met Sam during an afternoon break, when I'd agreed to take Erin out to the coffee shop. I breezed into Erin's apartment and noticed the young man sitting on her couch. Erin came right out of the bathroom wearing gray sweatpants that bagged over her fleshless legs. Her face was pale, and when she picked up her glasses, I realized that I usually saw her eyes through the lenses, which partly hid how sunken and weary they looked. She introduced the young man as Sam, whom she had met in her Partial program. He leaned over and kissed her gently before she and I left for our date.

The little café was crowded when we arrived, the atmosphere festive with the advent of Christmas. We hugged the owners, Tom and Judy, who invited us to stop by on Christmas Eve. Nearly all the other customers had left within minutes after I ordered Erin's large tea and my café Americano, and we settled into our favorite table against the wall, appreciating the quiet and privacy.

"I'm trying to have a friendship with Dad," she said. "We've been out three times lately, but I always feel sick afterwards."

I noticed that I didn't have that familiar self-satisfied reaction to any difficulty she had with Roger. I often felt redeemed when she had a problem with him, as if we were vying for the one Good Parent slot, or playing hot potato with the Bad Parent role.

"Sam also felt sick after meeting him, but Dr. Patton thinks my issues are with you." She paused, looking up from her tea, and added, "What mother and daughter don't have issues?"

One ear was on her, the other monitored my internal radar. I was surprised not to be feeling defensive or indignant at the psychiatrist's assumption.

"I want a more adult relationship with you," she continued. "You know, more like friends than mother-daughter."

Her eyes, so huge in that gaunt little face, pleaded with me. *See me as a Real Daughter, and not this sick, needy, dependent person I hate being and seeing you see me as.*

She said, "I want you to be able to come to me for support, too."

"We can work on that, honey," I replied, not wanting to burst this little bubble of imagined strength.

How could I even begin to think of looking for support from her? If she stumbles on her path, I will pick her up and carry her. But she can barely carry her own weight, much less help to carry mine.

Several days later, Erin came over to the house with Sam in tow. He hovered near her like an adoring golden retriever. All I saw was how badly she looked — her once thick and silky hair so thin that her scalp showed though, her skin pale, and her face and hands more gaunt than ever. She had been like this for so long, but I still had to override feeling repelled at the sight of my own daughter. And I don't see her naked. How can Sam possibly be attracted to her? I was aware of what a turn-around this was from the usual parental protectiveness — to wonder what he could see in her. There were still traces of beauty in what was left of her face, and she could be so sensitive and loving. But food and denying food came first.

"I'm making an appointment at Planned Parenthood to discuss birth control options. Sam doesn't want me to take birth control pills," she announced, as if this were a normal topic for her to broach.

I focused on the onions I was chopping, muzzling the voice that wanted to shout, *Are you crazy? How can you possibly think your body could get pregnant? Your body can barely keep you alive, much less grow a baby!*

After a few seconds I asked, "Have you had any periods?" knowing that she hadn't.

"A woman I knew at Remuda never had a period, and she had four children," she said, with a hint of defiance.

She really believes it's possible. She doesn't see how grotesque and freakish she looks. She fantasizes some normalcy for herself. I hate to even think it, but at times I wish she would just let go. I can't imagine why she is still alive, how her body does it.

Horrified at how she looked and horrified at myself that I could think of my own daughter dying as a relief, I stood with one foot on either side of an ever-widening chasm of grief. I was falling in no matter what. I couldn't imagine her living anything other than this strangulated version of a life. At least Sam was there for her.

Over the grilled cheese sandwiches I made him when he dropped by to talk, always hungry since there was nothing but cabbage and oatmeal in Erin's apartment, he told me about being beaten with boards by his father, who would tell him to "take it like a man." One of the beatings had knocked out his tooth. He said his mother didn't seem to notice the abuse. Tall and thin, with several chipped and missing teeth and a pleading smile, he seemed as vulnerable and emotionally starved as Erin was physically. Sam had been referred to Partial following discharge from the behavioral science unit for threatening suicide.

It was a cold January evening in 1999 when Sam called to tell me that Erin had cut herself while chopping carrots, and her index finger hadn't stopped bleeding. I drove down to pick them up to take her to the emergency room. After the admission paperwork, Erin was taken into the treatment area.

As soon as she was out of earshot, Sam started to talk. "I don't know what to do to help her. I want to fight this with her, but nothing I say or do makes any difference."

His green eyes were woeful, and there was a gap where his left incisor should have been. His shoulders looked especially bony through the short-sleeved T-shirt so inadequate on this cold mid-winter night. He seemed almost as pathetic and in need of protection as she did. But I appreciated his intent and the love he had for her. He needed rescuing himself, so where else could he feel like the strong one?

"You can't fight this for her, Sam. Believe me, we have been doing all that we can for years."

"I know I come in a distant second to food. She doesn't even know I'm there when she starts bingeing at night. She makes me sleep on the floor and won't give me a blanket or let me turn up the heat. She ate all the groceries I bought, but got mad when I wanted some of the oatmeal she'd saved to binge on."

Even as he complained about being mistreated by her, he vowed to take care of her: "I won't give up on her." I wondered if he thought that I had.

Maybe by "saving" her, he hoped to feel some of the strength and power he never had. But he was as helpless and hapless with her as he was with his parents.

Two hours after we'd arrived, Erin emerged smiling, with her newly stitched finger bound in gauze, and I drove them home. If only all her wounds were so easy to mend.

Erin and Sam arrived early for a planned visit on a Sunday afternoon. Sam had already given her an engagement ring, and I tried to suspend judgment about what could be "wrong" with him to want to marry her in this state. She couldn't have weighed more than 70 pounds.

It was a bright day and unusually warm for January, and I wanted to get outside while the sun was keeping the winter chill at bay. I invited Sam to walk to the BiLo with me to pick up a few of the groceries we needed for dinner, while Erin went to Walmart with Andrew. On our short walk we chatted about his ongoing concern for Erin's physical well-being and how devoted he was to helping her get better. He had cast himself as the white knight who wouldn't rest until he had rescued his fair maiden from the evil spell cast upon her. None of my cautionary words could dampen this fantasy in which he had a starring role.

At the market, I picked out broccoli, several heads of garlic, and a half-gallon of ice cream, and walked over to the express checkout line. As the groceries traveled along the belt toward the cash register, I opened my wallet to pay for the food. The billfold was empty. My mind went into rapid rewind as I stopped breathing. Had I spent anything since I put $80 in there yesterday? And then I remembered Erin sitting at the computer before we'd left, e-mailing Ariel. My purse had been on the floor beside her.

I felt sick to my stomach when I realized she had done it again. I refocused on the cashier and found two twenties where I keep a reserve stash folded under my driver's license. I took the change she handed back without looking at it, picked up the bags, and walked out of the store in a trance, hardly seeing Sam at my side. My mind raced as the familiar angry sadness flooded my body with adrenaline, clouding the otherwise sunny afternoon. I wanted to scream, jump up and down, or run as fast as I could. I told Sam what I thought had happened.

He read the anger in my face and said, "She's not responsible for what she does."

"Yes, she is!" I said, trying not to yell at him. "She may be out of control in her addiction, but she's still responsible for her behavior!"

I knew that the addiction possessed her when she stole, just like when she binged, but I refused to absolve her.

When Sam and I got home, I asked Erin to step into the living room, where we could be alone. I told her that money was missing from my wallet. She looked dumbfounded and befuddled. I had seen that look before.

As I looked into her eyes, I said, "I know you took it. How much did you take?"

"How much is missing?" she asked.

"A lot," I parried.

I knew better than to quote an exact amount.

"How much did you take?" I repeated.

"I don't know," she conceded.

"Where is it?" I asked, wondering if she had already spent it at Walmart.

"In my wallet."

She went over to where her jacket was draped on a chair, took her wallet out of the right front pocket, and handed me $30.

"That's not even close," I said with forced patience.

"Here," and she gave me another $20. "That's all I took for sure."

I was certain it wasn't, but decided to drop my end of the rope. It was a hollow victory, and a few more dollars meant nothing at this point.

"Please sit with me for a little while," she said as she looked at me with pleading, wet eyes. "I feel awful."

Drained by the atonement I had forced on her, I replied flatly, "I need some space right now."

Getting the money back was easy. Coaxing my heart out of its protective shell wasn't. She was pleading for my forgiveness, but I was still sore and tight with lingering anger and hurt. I didn't want to hurt her, but I needed time before I could embrace her with the love she wanted to feel. I went into the kitchen to be with Andrew, and Sam came into the living room to console her.

My anger dissipated quickly from that point, replaced by weary resignation. We had played this scene so many times, and even though I believed that, as Andrew reassured me later, I handled it well, I didn't feel good at all. I never did. Getting her to confess didn't solve anything. Though I felt compelled to wring an admission out of her, I didn't trust her not to steal again if the opportunity arose. Once more we realized that we had to be more vigilant when she was in the house, for her sake and for ours. I knew she didn't want or intend to violate me — she simply did what she did to feed her habit. Whether she intended to stab me or slipped, slicing me open by accident, I bled. I felt betrayed, yet I knew this had nothing to do with me. There was no answer or foolproof plan.

Two days later I answered the phone, barely able to make out the words through her sobs: "I'm so afraid of losing you. I feel so terrible about what I've done. I'm so ashamed. I love you so much. I don't want to lose you!"

"Honey, you will never lose me, no matter what. I love you. Nothing will ever change that," I said, pleading for her to believe me.

"How can you forgive me after all the times I have hurt you?" she sobbed.

"I just do," I said. "I may be hurt and angry, but that doesn't mean I don't love you."

"You and Andrew are so important to me. I don't ever want to lose you."

Her sobs started to soften, and she sounded less hysterical.

We'd had this exchange a hundred times. First, I'd treasure the moment. She loved me, and I loved her. No games. No power struggle. No unspoken accusations pushing through the words she said out loud. But then I'd remember all the times I'd held my ground with her behind a shield of anger, and I'd question myself. Was I too harsh? Was I trying to punish her, instead of just delivering the consequences she deserved and that I needed to get past feeling victimized once again?

Even though I was no longer angry and felt gratified by the remorse in her voice, I believed I had to hold her accountable. I'd argue inside my own head: It was not about revenge or blame, but about treating her as a whole human being. If there weren't any consequences for what she did in the throes of her addiction, then wasn't I conceding to that, as well? I refused to debase her by also surrendering all hope to her limitations.

Please, I prayed, *let there be some part of her that is a shining crescent of light not eclipsed by the disease.*

And then the final realization: as sensible as all that sounded, I had created an elaborate rationalization that helped me avoid admitting how hopeless and helpless she was. If she were responsible, then she could change. If she were not responsible, then it was out of her (and my) hands.

Several months later the home telephone rang as I was finishing my lunch and preparing for my afternoon sessions.

"I'm thinking of moving back to Chester County. I know I can get a job in construction down there. Erin wants to move, too. She's angry with all of you."

Suddenly he was allied with her, and we were the enemy. I was trying to make sense of this yet hold it at a distance — her anger with us, his passivity and perseverance, and how cruel and insensitive she could be. And now he wanted to move back to where he was so brutally abused and take his latest abuser with him. Except this time it was a 70-pound frail female instead of a 250-pound contractor.

I didn't expect that Erin would move. Even with all the support and sunshine at Chandler, she missed home and family. Shortly thereafter, Sam mysteriously evaporated from Erin's life and we never saw him again. Sam had stepped in as the surrogate savior and victim, mirroring the roles I resisted yet often felt. Seeing Erin alternately cling to him and abuse him with her addictive hoarding reinforced how sick she was, and helped me release any guilt I still had about her living on her own. I saw from a distance the conflicting parts of her that I struggled to reconcile — the part that felt sick and hopeless, the part that denied the reality of her condition, and the part that played out the addiction.

Rock-a-Bye Baby

If the world were only pain and
logic, who would want it?

MARY OLIVER

Erin's 23rd birthday, Thanksgiving, and Christmas all passed, with her impossibly more emaciated presence casting a shadow over our family celebrations. When she visited, she showed us drawings that weren't anything like the intricate and evocative creations hanging on our walls. Instead, they were either colored pen flowers and designs reminiscent of her pre-adolescent creations, or pastel, feathery angels as amorphous as her body had become. Did she long to return to the innocent freedom she felt before the eating disorder possessed her, or was she dreaming of the only future in which she could be free?

On February 6, the telephone rang as I was rinsing dishes after our evening meal. When I picked up and heard Erin's voice, I instinctively tensed up. But her voice was clear and sweet.

"When can I see you?" she asked.

This was a switch. Usually, I was the one who called or visited if we hadn't been in touch for a few days. Erin rarely called unless she was angry or apologetic. But this time, she seemed to simply want to be with me. I felt a wave of relief.

"I can pick you up during my break tomorrow, and we can have lunch together," I suggested.

It felt so easy, the way a mother and daughter connection was supposed to be.

The next afternoon at 1:15, I pulled up in front of Erin's apartment building. I watched her emerge from the front door, wearing pale blue sweatpants that bagged over her stick legs and a green plaid winter jacket that was several sizes too large. In her right hand she clutched her ever-present canvas tote bag. She walked slowly to the car, her expression wholly concentrated on the effort of lifting her legs.

As I opened the car door, Erin handed me her bag, and I noticed that she used both arms to pull herself up into the front seat of the Pathfinder. Though she had little weight to lift, her legs were no longer strong enough to make the step alone. When she turned in her seat to say hello, I saw tiny blue veins showing through skin stretched impossibly thinly over her cheekbones. I'd thought I was no longer capable of being shocked by her appearance, but I was wrong.

"Honey, you can't go on like this."

This was my code for suggesting it was time for her to be hospitalized again. I hadn't brought up hospitalization since the visit the past summer when Erin had been in the hospital. One of my visits coincided with her grandmother, Carol, coming to see Erin, as well. When Carol questioned why Erin and I were discussing another possible treatment facility, Erin told her about the harsh discipline she'd received from Roger, and despite Carol being upset, I was firm in defending how Erin could have been deeply affected by Roger's behavior. Erin was so grateful that I stood up to Carol.

At that point, Erin actually seemed relieved to have others in control and appeared receptive to the idea of entering a longer-term treatment program. But once out of the hospital she quickly returned to her old habits and refused to even con-sider the possibility of further treatment. Now, she looked even worse — thinner, weaker, paler — than she had when she'd been admitted seven months ago.

Picking up on my thinly veiled message, she replied quietly but firmly, "I don't want to go into the hospital again."

"Then you have to do something to take care of yourself," I responded.

My words sounded trite and obvious, like telling an alco-holic she had to stop hanging out in bars. But the shock of seeing Erin so deteriorated unleashed a torrent of protective, panicky love that drowned out the internal editor who usually framed every request in soothing therapist-speak. It was too late in the game for choosing words. I had to trust that the caring behind my bluntness came through.

"I think I want to be an art therapist who works with chil-dren," Erin suddenly announced, as if we'd been bouncing around career choices instead of discussing the desperate state of her health. Climbing Mount Everest seemed equally likely for her at this point. Still, I didn't want to snuff out that small, unexpected spark of a dream: Imagining a future beyond the next binge was more than I'd heard from her in months.

"That sounds like a wonderful goal to work toward, but first you'll have to take care of yourself," I repeated. My voice was soft and patient, but my mind was shrieking: *You're barely alive! How could you even imagine going to school, much less working with children?*

"I know," she said, as if she were prepared for that motherly reality check.

When we arrived at the house, I opened the kitchen cabinet and took out a can of minestrone.

"Do you have any frozen spinach?" Erin asked as she watched me open the can and stir the soup in a small pot.

Enacting a well-practiced ritual, I took a package of spinach out of the freezer, thawed it in the microwave, and drained it in a colander. Then she placed the steaming green strands in a bowl and mixed in a few flakes of canned tuna that she'd brought in her bag. I didn't protest: I knew that if I suggested anything more, even a few spoonfuls of soup, I would break the relaxed mood. Right now, nothing was more important than this gentle connection. No tension. No battling agendas.

The bright midday sun streamed in through the large west window, warming us as we sat at the kitchen table. Our silence felt peaceful, even sacred. Erin nibbled slowly at her meager lunch and sipped a large cup of herbal tea sweetened by two pink packets from her bag. As I ate my bowl of soup, I drank in the peace between us.

How beautiful her large green eyes are, like shimmering gems shining through the ruins of her body. As though she'd read my thought bubble, Erin stood up and disappeared into the bathroom to look in the large mirror.

"It's hard for me to see how bad I look," she said as she returned to the table.

Her voice was cheerful. As she walked toward me, I saw the sharp outline of her thighbones pushing against her sweatpants, and her sweatshirt hanging from wire-hanger shoulders. Maybe she really is helpless to change this, I thought. I had never heard my daughter show anything but veiled pride in her lack of flesh.

As I finished the last of my soup and put down my spoon, I saw that Erin was looking at me.

"Can I sit in your lap?" she asked.

Her voice was soft and high, like a little girl's. For years, I'd hated the feel of her body against mine. I regularly hugged her because I knew I should, but I dreaded the visceral reality of her knobby thinness against my soft flesh. This time, I didn't hesitate. She seemed so open and vulnerable, like a tiny, wounded bird. I pushed my chair back from the table and opened my arms. She settled herself into my lap and arranged her ribs against my chest.

As her head dropped onto my shoulder, she let out a breath and all but melted into my body. It was as though she'd been waiting forever to be enfolded by my arms again. I drank in the peace of being with my daughter without a struggle. The love between us ran clear, purified of the fear and anger that so often polluted our connection.

The dong of the university's carillon bell pulled me out of our shared, sweet silence. My first afternoon client was due to arrive in 30 minutes.

"I have to take you home, now, honey," I murmured.

I didn't want to let her go.

As we drove back to her apartment, she said, abruptly, "I'm so tired of the pain. I wish I could just die."

There were no tears or desperation in her voice, just a quiet, sad ring of truth. I felt a stab of dread and, at the same time, a kind of horrified understanding. The truth was that if I were

Erin, I wouldn't want to live either. I didn't know how she tolerated the deep ache of constant gnawing hunger, then the furious bingeing and purging, and then the endless counting of hours and days before she allowed herself to binge again. What could it be like to always be in pain, so weak that one could barely walk?

"I know I can't pray to Jesus to take me because that would be wrong," she went on softly. "He will release me in His time."

I recalled her attempted suicide seven years before as I listened to her careen between career dreams and death wishes. Nothing my daughter said or felt could surprise me anymore. So in this moment, I chose to linger in the afterglow of the tender hour we'd just shared.

After I pulled up to the curb in front of her apartment, Erin reached into her bag.

"I've got something for you," she said, and pulled out a white plush bear angel. It was a whimsical creature with satin ivory wings and a red nose.

"I want you to have this so that we are always connected in spirit," she said, her voice suddenly shy.

I noticed that her eyes were glistening. I didn't know what prompted this unexpected gift, but I felt a rush of gratitude: the miniature bear felt like the brush of an angelic wing on the brow of our shared sorrow. I also felt a distant prickle of hope: maybe she realized she needed to go into the hospital again.

I kissed her goodbye on the forehead, and she stepped gingerly out of the car. I pulled away slowly and struggled to shift emotional gears as I drove toward an afternoon of clients. My heart was still swimming in the tears I'd seen pooled in my daughter's eyes, and I was gripped by a sudden urge to turn the car around, burst through her apartment door and sweep her up once again into the safe, enveloping cocoon of my arms. I wanted to rock my baby. But I had to work.

At 10 that evening, the phone rang. Andrew picked up the extension next to our bed.

"It's for you," he said, handing me the phone.

It was Erin's disability caseworker.

"A friend found Erin unconscious in her apartment an hour ago," she said, her voice even but tense. "The ambulance has taken her to the hospital."

My heart jumped, but a part of me remained calm.

"Thanks for letting us know," I replied. "I'll call the hospital and find out what's happening."

I was able to keep my wits about me because Erin had survived this kind of emergency before — many times. I remembered the time she arrived for a scheduled inpatient stay in Pittsburgh, and her potassium levels had plunged to such a dangerously low point that the doctors couldn't understand how she remained alive, much less speak coherently. Countless times, I'd stopped by Erin's apartment wondering whether I would find her alive. But she was always there, her heart still faithfully beating despite the damage wreaked by her endless bingeing and purging. Bewilderingly, her body seemed built for endurance.

I dialed the emergency room; I knew the number by heart. "I'm Erin's mother. How is she?" This was before HIPAA regulations would have prohibited the staff from even acknowledging that my daughter was there, much less sharing information with me.

"She's still unconscious, but the doctor is with her," the nurse replied.

She didn't sound alarmed.

"Please call me if we need to come over," I said, and gave the nurse our telephone number.

Handing the phone back to Andrew to hang up, I thought, *Here we go again. Well, at least she's in the hospital where she'll get the care she needs.*

I turned off the light, but I had trouble sleeping.

Relax, I told myself. *They'll call if she gets worse.*

The next morning, the sky was clear and blue as I drove to the hospital after asking a colleague to post a sign on the office door in Corning saying that I wouldn't be in due to a family emergency. I picked Jocelyn up from the high school — Jenna and Ariel were both in college 250 miles away, and Zane had a class at the local university. As we entered the building, the hospital chaplain was waiting for me in the corridor.

"Mrs. Seubert?"

I nodded, instinctively looking away from his kind eyes. My heart began to pound. *No, she can't be. Maybe he thinks I need some spiritual guidance as Erin slowly pulls through. After all, that's his job.*

But as he led me to the intensive care waiting room, he was quiet. A moment later our family doctor was standing next to us. I forced myself to look at him.

"She's gone," he said quietly.

"No!" My voice was strangled by a sob. "No!" *She always pulls through!*

Over the doctor's shoulder, I saw Andrew burst through the door.

"They called just after you left the house," he said, his voice catching.

We fell into each other's arms. After a few minutes, the doctor gently guided all three of us to Erin's bedside.

"She never regained consciousness," he said.

There Erin lay, covered by a thin hospital gown, still connected by tubes and wires to the gray, blinking heart monitor and IV pole. Her eyes were closed, her expression calm. For a few timeless moments I watched over my daughter's still body, finally released from its torments.

Your struggle is over, I thought. *You got your wish, and you're free.*

I, too, was free. Freed from a mother's fearful helplessness. And alive, but irrevocably aware of the emptiness in my arms.

26

Riptide

Grace means you're in a different
universe from where you had been
stuck, when you had absolutely
no way to get there on your own.

ANNE LAMOTT

Andrew and I were seated around the dining room table with
our friends Jill and Ted, the remains of Sunday brunch piled to
one side. Erin had died three years earlier, and though I missed
her terribly and was reminded of her countless times a day, I'd
embraced my life with gratitude and rested in the relief that she
was out of pain — a relief that was still tinged with stabbing
guilt about what I could have or should have done and been.

"How is Ben doing?" I asked Jill and Ted.

We knew that their younger son had battled suicidal depression during the past year while away at college.

"He's back at school after taking a semester off," Jill replied.

An experienced psychologist whose intelligence and sensitivity showed through her large brown eyes, Jill continued, "The medications seem to be working, and he's finally bouncing back from the break-up with his girlfriend. I still worry about him, but I need to remember that he's an adult now. It's awful to feel so helpless. And it's so darned hard to let go."

"Believe me," I replied, "I know."

Jill's eyes glistened with tears. "I know you do."

She looked up, pausing, and then said, "Did I ever tell you about the time Ben and I nearly drowned?"

"No," I replied, curious about where this was going. "What happened?"

"We were spending a week at the shore with the boys. Ben was nine and Jon was twelve. Ben and I were having a great time in the water when I felt a powerful current pulling me away from shore. I realized that we must be caught in a riptide. We started yelling and waving at the people on the beach, who were getting farther and father away. A few people waved back, probably thinking we were just fooling around. 'Swim as hard as you can!' I yelled at Ben, but we were being carried farther and farther from the beach. 'Don't give up!' I screamed to him over and over, even though I was sure we were going to die."

She paused, as if she had to catch her breath the way she did in the water.

"I was never more helpless and afraid. If I had been alone, I might have given up. Ben thought that I saved him, but actually the wind that pushed us down the beach, along with our own swimming, saved us."

"What a close call!" I exclaimed, thinking that this was the end of the story.

"It was, but that was nothing like the terror I felt when Ben was depressed. I did what I could to help him, but months went by and he wasn't pulling out of it. Finally I realized what I'd been frightened of when we were out there in the ocean, caught in the riptide. What I realized was I didn't have the power to save another person, even if he were my son."

She drew a deep breath.

"Even if I would trade my life for his in a heartbeat."

I didn't *choose* not to save Erin. I *couldn't* save her.

I felt relief course through my body. But Jill had still more to say.

"During those months of Ben's depression, I realized that I couldn't live my son's life, much less know the demons within him," she said, standing up and holding the back of her chair. "I finally realized that I couldn't be there for him, really there for him, unless I admitted to myself that he could die. And I had to keep living my own life or I would stop being me. My own anxiety, stress, and terror kept me away from my son, and away from myself."

As she looked into my eyes, I felt a gentle tide of absolution wash over me. I stood up and hugged her, my heart floating in a sea of grace.

That evening I climbed into the hot tub on our snow-covered patio, a glass of shiraz in hand. The sky was black and studded with stars, and I watched the tiny blinking light of a plane cross the dark expanse above me. I could see Andrew through the large window behind the spa as he stood at the stove, finishing a risotto for our dinner before coming out to join me. The night air was crisp and cold against my face, and I welcomed the heat penetrating my body. Sipping my wine, I was filled with gratitude for the blessings of my senses. I beamed my love to Erin among the stars, grateful for the life that had passed through mine like the plane's flight, speeding toward a destination I could not know or change, only witness.

Pietà

There are no guarantees. From
the viewpoint of fear, none are
strong enough. From the viewpoint
of love, none are necessary.

EMMANUEL

When Andrew and I were in Italy four years after Erin's death, one of the most memorable stops on our tour was the Museo dell'Opera del Duomo in Florence. As our small tour group followed our guide through the extensive collection of pre-Renaissance and Renaissance sculpture, I stopped, as if frozen in place, staring at Michelangelo's unfinished and final Pietà. Unexpected tears streamed down my cheeks as I gazed at the expression on Christ's face, his lifeless body draped across Mary's lap. Andrew had moved on with our companions to another exhibit, while I stood, transfixed by how this centuries-old piece of marble could mirror feelings I didn't even know how to articulate. I pulled myself out of the trance to find Andrew, who had moved on to the next room, to bring him back, hoping he could see what had cast such a spell on me.

"It's an expression of sweet relief," he reflected, "as if he's saying the suffering is finally over."

That was it. For all the pain of witnessing her son's suffering, Mary was at peace. The worst was over, and she knew her son had been released.

In *A New Earth*, Eckhart Tolle writes of the importance of surrender, the surrender that releases us from fighting with what is. Just as Jill had said about surviving a riptide, if you swim against the current, you simply become exhausted and are pulled under more quickly. I fought for years against Erin's disease, against the parts of her that seemed wedded to her disease, and against the possibility that I might be at fault. I didn't know how to find peace without figuring out what I could do, or she should do, to make "what was" what I wanted. I swung on the pendulum between trying to control and giving up, knowing little of surrender and nothing of peace, believing that only after my child was able to gnaw her way through the ropes that bound her could I be whole and happy again. There wasn't a single, discreet moment when I held up the white flag and let go. I had to grieve for what would not be, in order to be with what was.

As I stood in front of that Pietà in Florence, I became one with all mothers throughout time who had suffered and grieved, cradled in the arms of the Great Heart that is able to hold us together, knows our pain, and gives us the strength to go on. I was both the mother and the child, the sweetness of suffering relieved encompassing us all. I felt a part of a community anointed by pain and blessed by gratitude for the beauty and boundlessness of the compassion that contains every one of us. I was both humbled and held up, saddened and sanctified, a small yet significant drop in an ocean of love.

ACKNOWLEDGMENTS

Without the wonderful support of a number of skilled and compassionate readers, coaches, editors, and friends, I might never have had the courage to complete this project. Enormous gratitude goes to the following who were active and essential at various stages of the process:

Cindy Barrilleaux, my first writing midwife and coach whose wise, patient, and loving guidance was invaluable through the early stages of this manuscript; Marion Sandmaier, who masterfully edited several chapters; Ed Schuster, for insightful content editing and steadfast encouragement; Rhonda Morton, for astute copy and content editing; Constance Sullivan-Blum, for reading, inspiring the title, and for being such a good friend; Judith Sornberger, for friendship and the class that convinced me I could write.

Special thanks to Jen Hale at ECW Press for believing in my manuscript and for her perceptive and sensitive attention to impact on others and flow.

To the Lifelong Gestalt group and our beloved mentor and fellow member, Clifford Smith, with whom there is no doubt we are all in this together, I can't thank you all enough for the experience of how it should always be.

Thanks to Wendy Moran, Alycia Chambers, and Rob Gentry, for sharing their own experiences and for their loving presence in my life. To Tom Bernard, who is greatly missed by us all. And to Margaret Launius, whose friendship, love, and humor will live forever.

Enormous gratitude to Carolyn Hodges Chaffee for 20 years of support and friendship, and to the devoted Nutrition Clinic staff for making the annual Erin Leah Memorial Conference such a success year after year.

I also thank the parents who kindly and courageously shared their stories with me. Though I didn't include that material, it was essential to my understanding of how universal our struggles can be.

Words are inadequate to express the love and gratitude I feel for the unending support and encouragement from my beloved husband, Andrew. No one has done more to help me heal, persevere, and know that I am loved. To Zane of the open and forgiving heart — you are an inspiration. And finally, to my amazingly wise, strong, and beautiful daughters — Jenna, Ariel, and Jocelyn — I couldn't be more blessed to love and be loved by you.

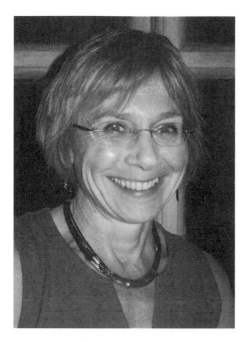

Barbara Hale-Seubert is a
psychotherapist in practice with
her husband, Andrew, and is the
parent of three surviving daughters
and a stepson. She lives in
Mansfield, Pennsylvania.